ARE YOU AFRAID TO QUIT? . . .

HERE ARE THE ANSWERS YOU'RE LOOKING FOR.

Q: Will the program be hard to follow?
A: No. You will be able to stop smoking in thirty days—without weight gain.

Q: Will the recommended micronutrients be expensive?
A: No. And they are readily available at any health food store.

Q: How will I get started in the morning without the first cigarette?
A: The supplements you take will give you that "feel good" sensation you get from nicotine.

Q: When I tried to quit smoking before, I got really hungry.
A: No more hunger pangs when you follow the Cellular Nutrition Program.

Q: How do I avoid the weight gain?
A: The program is designed to help you STOP SMOKING, STAY SKINNY!

D1491002

STOP SMOKING, STAY SKINNY

DR. JOSEPH T. MARTORANO
CARMEL BERMAN REINGOLD

AVON BOOKS ◆ NEW YORK

The ideas, procedures, and suggestions in this book are intended to supplement, not replace, the medical advice of a trained medical professional. All matters regarding your health require medical supervision. Consult your physician before adopting the suggestions in this book, as well as any condition that may require diagnosis or medical attention. The author and publisher disclaim any liability arising directly or indirectly from the use of this book.

AVON BOOKS
A division of
The Hearst Corporation
1350 Avenue of the Americas
New York, New York 10019

Copyright © 1998 by Dr. Joseph T. Martorano and Carmel Berman Reingold
Published by arrangement with the authors
Visit our website at http://www.AvonBooks.com
Library of Congress Catalog Card Number: 97-94078
ISBN: 0-380-79496-9

First Avon Books Printing: February 1998

AVON TRADEMARK REG. U.S. PAT. OFF. AND IN OTHER COUNTRIES, MARCA REGISTRADA, HECHO EN U.S.A.

Printed in the U.S.A.

WCD 10 9 8 7 6 5 4 3

CONTENTS

STOP SMOKING, STAY SKINNY

ONE

WHEN YOU STARTED SMOKING

Almost everyone can trace their smoking habit to the very day they started:

- *"I was fifteen and going to this really big party at my cousin's house. She lived in Chicago and I lived in a small town. I just knew that her friends were happening people. When someone offered me a cigarette I took it. I didn't want to be different."*
- *"I was studying for finals at Bob's house. His parents smoked, and they didn't mind if Bob and I took a cigarette."*
- *"I was starting a new job . . . A cigarette made me feel I could handle it."*
- *"All the guys in my dorm smoked."*

Those are some of the comments, and we also heard:

- " . . . *I feel more confident with a cigarette . . .* "
- " . . . *I feel calm when I smoke . . .* "
- " . . . *I have more energy when I smoke . . .* "
- " . . . *Cigarettes give me something to do with my hands . . .* "

Okay, smoking was cool, smoking was hip, smoking was neat.

Everything that was said was true. If smoking tasted like castor oil, or made you feel as though you had just swallowed ten hot chili peppers, you wouldn't continue smoking—nobody would.

What makes a drug or food tempting is that it tastes good and makes you feel good. That's why people smoke and eat chocolate éclairs.

BUT IT DIDN'T MAKE YOU FEEL GOOD AT FIRST

An interesting fact: Maybe you tried to hide it from your friends, but that first cigarette did not make you feel good. It probably made you feel nauseated, a little dizzy, high—but not in a good way.

You didn't let on about this to anyone. You thought you might feel better after a second cigarette, or a third, so you kept on smoking, and sure enough, by the third cigarette you felt great—and by that third cigarette you were also hooked. Nobody is born loving a cigarette. But it takes a very short time to become a cigarette addict, a tobacco junkie. And cigarettes have an even more potent hook: They're legal and they can help keep you skinny.

WHY YOU STILL SMOKE: PERSONAL REASONS

Okay, why are you still smoking? You know the facts—you're no dummy.

"Still smoking?" someone asks.

"I need a cigarette to stay calm," is one answer.

"Cigarettes are like uppers for me," is another.

"I work a long day—cigarettes give me energy to get me through it."

And then there's the most potent reason of all: ***"I tried quitting and gained ten pounds."***

"My friend Gerald quit. He gained fifteen pounds and he hasn't been able to get it off."

And, here's the real biggie:

"I'D RATHER BE DEAD THAN FAT!"

If you have ever said that, you're not alone. A whole lot of people say that, but do they mean it? *Do you?* We don't think anyone really wants to die—especially for such a frivolous cause.

Sure, it would be great to have a body like one of those models in *Vogue* or *GQ*—but to die for it? We don't think so, and neither do you—not really.

The other response often heard was: *"I am going to stop smoking . . . someday."*

When?

"After I become an editor. You should see the women at the magazine—they're all skinny."

"There's this girl I'm interested in . . . I don't think she digs chubby guys."

"After I get engaged."

"After I get married . . . I want to walk down the aisle in a size four wedding dress . . . "

"After my vacation! I'm going to Club Med and I don't want to look fat in a bathing suit . . . "

Sure, you'll quit smoking *sometime*. As Saint Augustine supposedly prayed: "Make me good, O Lord, but not just yet."

Or maybe you really decided to give up smoking, and you actually did it—a few times. But without your cigarettes you felt depressed, nervous, edgy—and to make it even worse, instead of reaching for a cigarette, you stretched your hand out for a candy bar—a whole lot of candy bars.

"It's not fair," we heard more than once. *"I stopped smoking and I felt terrible. I thought* not *smoking was supposed to make me feel better. Great. But I was exhausted. Then I got on the scale!"*

That isn't true for everyone—some lucky souls quit smoking and never gain an ounce. There are people who never have a bad hair day, either. But practically everyone gains weight right after they quit. First, because they substitute sweets and fats for cigarettes, and second, because their metabolism functions differently. What to do? You want to do the right thing for your health, but cigarettes make you feel better—and they keep you thin. Life without cigarettes? Maybe it's not worth living after all.

A DIRTY LITTLE SECRET

You work or you go to school. You pass tests, you complete job or school assignments. You're up for a promotion, a raise, a degree. Why does such a responsible person find it so hard to quit smoking?

The answer: Smoking is more than a habit. It is an addiction.

Everyone knows that heroin, coke, crack, and cocaine are addictive, but cigarettes? Very addictive, and that fact was only recently revealed and recognized—even admitted by one cigarette company.

Oh, sure, there are still certain types out there— some cigarette manufacturers and a few politicians— who say: "Cigarettes may be addictive, but only if you're the addictive type."

That means that nearly fifty million Americans who smoke are addictive types.

SAY GOOD-BYE TO GUILT

Okay, now you know: You're an addict, a nicotine addict.

"Addict," a two-pack-a-day smoker said. "That word makes me feel bad, *guilty*."

We heard the word *guilty* from many smokers—and it was the word, and the feelings it engendered, that caused many people to continue smoking.

Have you ever said, "I'm weak, I can't give up cigarettes"?

That is followed by guilt about not being able to kick a dangerous habit, and then comes: "I'm going to die eventually anyway. I may as well continue smoking."

But no one starts out being addicted to tobacco. *Your addiction is not your fault.* You became addicted without realizing that it was happening. You bought or were given a drug that is legally obtainable. And despite all the warnings written on every pack, cigarettes are easily and cheaply available.

"Everyone smokes."

"My grandfather lived to be ninety and he smoked."

Those are some of the rationales for smoking. When you started, it seemed as though a friendly hand was held out to you, a hand that led you down a dangerous path lined with cigarettes.

Try to remember how you felt when you smoked that first cigarette. You smoked it—but you felt like throwing up. But you were urged on—by friends, by custom, by ads that made smoking seem glamorous and fashionable, and finally by the way nicotine made you feel once you became accustomed to cigarettes. You were led gently into a trap, but now it's up to you to get out of it.

Do you feel as though you're all thumbs when you're not smoking?

Place a dish of beautiful small stones on your desk in a shallow dish. When you feel nervous, take a stone or two and clasp them between your hands, or toss them from hand to hand. The smooth, black river stones from Japan are great for this.

WHY AM I STILL SMOKING?

It's hard to quit smoking because nicotine affects the body in seemingly positive ways: Your metabolism works faster, which helps calories burn up; your blood sugar goes up and you get an extra burst of energy. Two glands—the hypothalamus and the adrenal—are affected.

Here's what happens to you physically and emotionally when you smoke, and when you try to quit smoking:

Nicotine stimulates the hypothalamus in the brain, raising the blood sugar level. The result is that you feel relaxed and you're not hungry.

When you quit smoking, the stimulation to the hypothalamus is withdrawn. The result is that your blood sugar takes a steep drop. This creates hunger pangs—especially for something sweet—and because you're doing your best not to reach for a chocolate bar, you become anxious and strung out.

Nicotine also stimulates the adrenal gland. That extra jolt of adrenaline courses through your system and lessens your appetite while giving your energy level a boost.

Nicotine also speeds up your metabolism, burning fuel (food and calories) more quickly. This keeps your weight down.

To experience all that, the amount of cigarettes you need increases. Maybe a few cigarettes made you feel good when you first started smoking, but as your body became accustomed to the effects of nicotine, you need more and still more cigarettes to feel quick, and smart, and high, and energized, and you need even more cigarettes to help you stay thin.

Now you're trying to quit smoking. You've heard all the bad news about cigarettes; maybe you've even seen some scary examples of what smoking can do. But without your nicotine fix, you're anxious, so rattled that you can't do your job properly. You're tired a lot of the time, and on top of that, you're hungry all the time.

IF NICOTINE MAKES ME FEEL SO GOOD, THEN WHY . . .

Why give up cigarettes? Without trying to soft-pedal the facts, here's why:

- People who smoke die fifteen years earlier than people who don't. That's 5,475 days lost from a life.
- Half a million Americans die each year of smoking-related illnesses.
- Millions more who smoke become victims of a variety of cancers, heart disease, high blood pressure, and emphysema.

And while Violetta dies glamorously in *La Traviata* of lung disease while wearing a ball gown and singing an aria, life is not an opera, and tobacco-related deaths and illnesses are a painful way to go.

THE HIGH THAT DOESN'T LAST

If you've been smoking for a while, you may be aware of another fact: The few cigarettes that gave you a high when you first started no longer have that same effect. The few cigarettes that originally stimulated often become depressants—unless you smoke more. Now you need a pack or more to get that *up* feeling.

LET'S GO BACK

Remember the way you felt when you first started smoking? You had more energy, you were stimulated when that was what you needed, and yet you also became calm when that was called for. All those good feelings and you kept your weight down. If only you could feel *that* good again—but without cigarettes.

CELLULAR NUTRITION

Now, thanks to Cellular Nutrition, we believe that you can feel as good as you did when you first started smoking, and you'll keep your weight down *without cigarettes*.

And if overweight is a problem even though you smoke, Cellular Nutrition can help you *get your weight down* as well as *keep it down*.

What is Cellular Nutrition? It's the absolute cutting edge of natural-oriented therapy that uses the latest information obtained through biochemical research to keep the body functioning at a healthy level.

THE CELL STORY

Before we tell you about Cellular Nutrition, here's an abbreviated course on the human cell right out of Biology 101.

Your body, and particularly your brain, is made up of cells. We are complex organisms, almost beyond our ability to picture. Recently neuroscientists revised their estimate of the number of cells in the human brain from an incredible twelve billion to a more staggering trillion cells.

Many years ago, Jules Hirsch, a brilliant scientist and researcher at Rockefeller University, explained that many people suffer from *hypertropic obesity*, wherein there is simply too much fat crammed into cells. To get past this, help is needed to speed the transport of fat through the cells.

Every cell in the body contains an element called *mitochondria*. The mitochondria are each cell's engine—the motor that keeps the cell going. If the mitochondria do not work properly, your cells bump along like an old car—not too healthy, maybe just getting by, holding on to fat.

DO YOU HAVE A MITOCHONDRIA PROBLEM?

Do you feel tired many mornings even after a full night's sleep? Maybe you catch colds often, and many of the foods you eat just don't seem to agree with you. If this sounds familiar, see your doctor. If the doctor doesn't find anything wrong, your problem may be sluggish cells.

Until now, when your body cried out for help, you reached for a cigarette. A few drags, a few more drags, maybe even a second cigarette quickly followed the first. The cigarettes raised your blood sugar and you felt better—for a short time. But the more you smoked, the more you needed that nicotine fix to get your blood sugar going. That's another downside to smoking: you need increasingly more nicotine to feel good.

Now you can turn things around and improve the condition of your cells. It's important to treat your cells *before* they accumulate too much fat. Once the mitochondria are working at a proper pace, you will have more energy, your blood sugar will be kept at an even keel so that you're not always hungry, and your metabolism will work to burn up calories.

THE PROGRAM

All this can be accomplished through Cellular Nutrition, which uses micronutrients and phytochemicals to get those mitochondrial engines humming.

As you smoke, nicotine pumps adrenaline into your system, giving you a surge of energy. By substituting micronutrients for cigarettes, you can stimulate the mitochondria, which then provide a more even flow of natural energy from better-functioning cells. Micronutrients also help repair the cells that have been ravaged by cigarettes and at the same time can help speed up the metabolism. A lethargic metabolism can be a source of weight gain.

When the micronutrients and phytochemicals copy the good effects of nicotine without the dangers, you'll have more energy, be better able to concentrate, enjoy a sense of·calm, and *stay skinny*—all that without having to smoke a single cigarette!

And if smoking did not do enough to control your weight, Cellular Nutrition may be the answer. If you're afraid to give up cigarettes because you believe that without smoking you would be even heavier, take heart—the Cellular Nutrition Program may help you lose weight even as you quit smoking.

WILL CELLULAR NUTRITION HELP ME?

Unfortunately, no program works for everyone. This is as true for conventional medical methods as it is for the less conventional kind. Before you embark on any lifestyle change involving your health, talk to your doctor.

"I'LL THINK ABOUT IT TOMORROW"

Scarlett O'Hara became famous for the oft-repeated phrase "I'll think about it tomorrow."

Scarlett could afford to do that, but can you? Every day that you continue smoking makes it that much harder to give up the habit.

In ancient times many people believed that a person could be possessed by the Devil. Today, there are devils of a different sort that can lay waste to a body. An addiction to drugs—and we know that cigarettes fall in that category—can be a destructive force that you have to battle. Working to give up smoking is a struggle—

but it's a struggle that's worth making because smoking can not only harm you, it can also harm the people you love. If you become ill, think how your family and friends will be hurt, and remember, too, that second-hand smoke is definitely a danger to the people around you. Be hopeful and be patient. Very few people can go cold turkey when giving up smoking, but you can arrive at a cigarette-free life in time. So take a deep breath and take the plunge. Start on the "Stop Smoking, Stay Skinny" plan today. You'll find it a lot easier than you thought it would be.

TWO

SEND IN THE SUBSTITUTES

Now that you understand why you smoke—and the reasons for your nicotine cravings—we hope that you have said good-bye to every last residue of guilt. With all those negative emotions out of the way, you can move forward. Thanks to the latest findings, and the way those findings have been incorporated into the Cellular Nutrition Program, you can now substitute healthy alternatives to cigarettes. These alternatives are the micronutrients that will mimic the feel-good effects of nicotine without endangering your health or life.

When we get to this point in talking about the Cellular Nutrition Program, we can't go on without being interrupted by questions.

Because you're probably sitting there, reading this book, with the very same questions on your mind, we will answer your questions first.

Q: Will this program be hard to follow?

A: No!

Q: But I really need that first cigarette in the morning to feel alert. Will those micronutrients help me get going?

A: They should give you lots of energy.

Q: When I tried to quit smoking before, I got really hungry.

A: No more hunger pangs when you follow the Cellular Nutrition Program.

Q: I know cigarettes are bad for me, and this may sound silly, but I don't want to get fat. What about that?

A: That doesn't sound silly to us. We understand how important that is to you, and what an important part weight plays in many facets of life today: social, business, and personal assessment of self.

We are never impatient with people who balance the dangers of smoking against the problem of weight gain. It's too bad that today's value system places so much importance on being thin. This may not be laudable, but it is the way things are, and we believe in working with what is—not what we would like it to be.

Now we can go on to tell you about the micronutrients in the Cellular Nutrition Program.

**What brings on a terrible craving
for cigarettes?**

*That 3:00 P.M. container of coffee, perhaps?
Break the association! Drink herbal tea or eat
an apple or pear. If you're home, peel the fruit
first—that keeps both hands occupied and too
busy to reach for a cigarette.*

THE MICRONUTRIENTS

This is where the micronutrients come into play.
Micronutrients are a minimal amount of a nutrient that
can effect changes in the cells of the body. They can
stimulate mitochondrial energy production and relieve
the stress of oxidation. Here are the micronutrients recommended for the program, and a description of what
each can do for you.

L-Carnitine . . . *What It Does:*
Carnitine is an amino acid that moves fatty acids
across the membrane of the cell and into the mitochondria.

This nutrient stimulates fat metabolism and works
within the cells to produce energy.

As your energy levels rise, your body burns fuel—
calories—more quickly.

Robert Crayon, the leading expert in L-carnitine

research, recommends that this micronutrient be purchased in *tartrate* form.

Chromium Picolinate . . . *What It Does:*

This has long been a favorite of movie stars and supermodels for whom remaining thin is a career necessity. Chromium picolinate normalizes blood sugar levels and makes the insulin your body produces behave more efficiently. The result is that you're not always hungry, and your cravings for sin foods such as chocolate truffles and ice cream are diminished. The good news continues: Chromium picolinate also metabolizes fat. This means that while you lose fat (not weight), you gain muscle. The result: a trimmer body.

Coenzyme 10 . . . *What It Does:*

A study conducted in Belgium indicated that many obese patients were totally deficient in this nutrient, which helps the body emulsify fat.

Coenzyme 10 also works with the mitochondria to produce energy, and as with L-carnitine, as your energy levels rise, your body burns up calories more quickly.

This nutrient also acts as an antioxidant—an important plus for smokers whose cells may have been damaged by nicotine.

Coenzyme 10 is frequently prescribed in Europe by doctors practicing conventional medicine.

The rest of the world knows about coenzyme 10. Fifteen million Japanese men take it every day for energy, for cardiovascular health, and to aid in weight loss.

Ginkgo Biloba . . . *What It Does:*

Ginkgo Biloba comes from the ginkgo tree with the pretty, fan-shaped leaves. They're so pretty that ginkgo leaves are used frequently as a design element in gold jewelry. In this case, pretty is as pretty does. The ginkgo tree is seen on many city sidewalks because it is one tree that is resistant to pollution.

You won't be munching on leaves, just taking a capsule that contains a concentrated ginkgo extract that has achieved popularity in Germany as an aid to circulation.

As you move away from cigarettes, ginkgo biloba can provide the energy previously obtained from nicotine. Ginkgo biloba also helps counteract depression, and it acts as an antioxidant.

Lecithin . . . *What It Does:*

Lecithin is an emulsifier, which means that it works within each cell to help fats emulsify with the cell's water base. This keeps the fat liquid and helps the fat keep moving. Lecithin is found in every cell, and acts as a natural diuretic—helping rid the body of excess water, which can create a bloated feeling and bloated look.

If you look at the list of ingredients on any box of chocolates, you will see lecithin. No, you can't eat chocolates instead of taking lecithin capsules, but the ingredient that gives chocolate that lovely, smooth texture can also do good things for you.

B Vitamins . . . *What They Do:*

The B vitamins are great stuff. They help metabolize fat by releasing energy from food. The Bs also relieve stress, and they're a big help when you experience the fatigue that hits when you're trying to stop smoking. B vitamins are more potent together than when used separately.

When taking a B complex capsule, check the label to make sure that it contains every important B. Here's what to look for: vitamin B_1, which may be listed as thiamine; B_2, as riboflavin; B_3, as niacin. Other important Bs are: pantothenic acid, biotin, folic acid, B_{12}, and B_6.

Additional Bs are choline and inositol, but don't fret if they're not in your B-complex capsule, because they're in lecithin.

It's the weekend and you're dying for a cigarette.

Go immediately to some place where smoking is not allowed: a museum, movie, department store. It's healthier to shop than it is to smoke, and you'll be saving so much money when you don't buy cigarettes that you'll be able to indulge in the store!

Phytochemicals: Herbs, Vegetables, Fruits

Phytochemicals are plant-derived nutrients that can contribute to health by creating favorable cellular change. A familiar example of phytochemical-rich food is the family of cruciferous vegetables, including broccoli, cauliflower, brussels sprouts, and kale.

Cruciferous vegetables are known to act as a preventative against cancer. And there are phytochemicals you can lean on when you quit smoking. They are:

GARLIC: lowers blood pressure and relieves stress and anxiety that may hit you when you're trying to quit smoking. Garlic also lowers blood sugar, and acts as an antioxidant.

Use the garlic you buy at the greengrocer rather than the supplement, which may or may not have side effects.

GINGER: soothes the nerves and settles the stomach. Use ginger root, which can be bought from the greengrocer, rather than powdered ginger, and if you're yearning for a sweet—have one or two pieces of candied ginger.

GREEN TEA: a favorite beverage in Japan, the best of which is used in the elegant tea ceremony. Green tea is prepared from the unfermented leaves of the tea plant—which explains why it's green, rather than the familiar black of most tea leaves.

Drink green tea rather than taking green tea supplements. It's an enjoyable beverage, and a great way to become wide-awake in the morning. If you don't think you can start your day without a cigarette, brew a pot of green tea. You'll experience a pleasant high, and the tea will also help keep your blood sugar level.

HOW TO TAKE MICRONUTRIENTS AND PHYTOCHEMICALS

We'll give you directions as to how and when to take micronutrients and phytochemicals. You should not gulp pills and capsules by the handful—that's not how it works.

Cellular Nutrition is a very precise program. You have to take the right amounts of highly specific micronutrients at specific times to effect internal cellular changes that will empower your cells to separate out from the effects of nicotine.

However, *before* starting on the program, talk to your doctor. Many physicians are becoming more sympathetic to alternative methods, and some HMOs are offering coverage for consulting alternative medical practitioners.

Going to a restaurant that has a smoking section?

Make sure that you reserve a table in the non-smoking room.

THREE

PSYCHOLOGICALLY SPEAKING

To quit smoking, you have to want to quit smoking. The first thing to do is to look within and come to terms with the real reasons you smoke, and why you continue to do so. Quitting is not easy.

Fifty-seven percent of the thousand people interviewed by the Addiction Research Foundation in Toronto said that giving up cigarettes would be harder for them than giving up alcohol or any other drug.

Many smokers, aware of the dangers of smoking, say, "I know all that, but I'm still having trouble. Do you think I can ever quit smoking?"

The answer is a loud YES. Your desire to smoke is triggered by an underlying physiological need, and Cellular Nutrition will help you cope with that aspect. But coupled with that physical craving are the psychological demands of your mind, and Dr. Martorano's Five-Step Plan offers important assistance.

23

The plan was originally created by Dr. Martorano for his best-selling book *Beyond Negative Thinking,* and it has been adapted to the needs of those who wish to stop smoking and control their weight at the same time.

Based on cutting-edge cognitive therapy, the plan will show you how to cope with the thoughts and inner speech that drive you to reach for a cigarette.

The Five-Step Plan uses the psychological approach that asks, "What are you thinking?" rather than "What are you feeling?" The plan will help you access your thoughts, and will show you how to change those thoughts in ways that will improve your life. Here are the basics of the plan:

FIVE STEPS

1. *Listening In.* Training to hear yourself thinking.
2. *Underlining.* Selecting the specific words in your internal dialogue that are detrimental to you and your own best interests.
3. *Stopping.* Shutting off the negative words in your internal thought speech.
4. *Switching.* Interrupting harmful inner speech and substituting positive internal voices.
5. *Reorienting.* Changing the thrust of your thinking to an active, problem-solving mode.

Listening In. Do you reach for a cigarette automatically? Or does a voice within say, "I want a cigarette *now*"? If your mind goes on automatic pilot whenever you reach for a cigarette, you must gradually learn to stop and think before taking that cigarette. Automatic won't do—pay attention to what is in your mind before you give in to that craving for a cigarette.

Underlining means selecting the specific words in your internal dialogue that are destructive to you. As you Listen In to your thoughts, some words will soon stand out as culprits. Underline them so that they become obvious to you. Once you have Underlined the words, you can act to change them constructively.

Now you've started listening . . . What is your inner voice saying? Is it "I want a cigarette" or "I need a cigarette" or "I must have a cigarette"?

Want, need, must have . . . Do you really intend to give up power so easily?

Underlining builds very closely on Listening In. When you practiced Listening, you became aware of what your inner speech was like. Now, with Underlining, you'll be highlighting the deadly words and phrases that poison your thoughts. The positive parts of your thinking, the thoughts that bolster you, don't need any attention. They're doing their job. What you need to concentrate on are the messages you don't need to hear.

Underlining will put you into touch with your own weak thoughts. Suppose you're Listening In and you hear your inner voice state, "I'm *hopeless*. I'll never be able to quit smoking." Immediately underline "hopeless." That term (the inner words in your mind) makes you feel exactly that way. It certainly does not serve any positive purpose.

Your thinking has done you a disservice. You have

been victimized by your own put-down. A damaging area, this. In the put-down, your inner voice sent you subtle, failure-provoking messages that caused you to feel weak or immature. Be on the lookout for them. Underline them. Just the existence of that thought in your mind, "hopeless," causes you to feel less of a person. It may seem too simple a technique to you right now; but if you do not think that thought, you will feel more effectual.

You can become a winner in the contest with your thoughts. You now have two valuable techniques that build on each other to help you. As you train yourself to use them, they'll become increasingly effective, and you'll find yourself gaining confidence in situations that used to throw you.

Stopping . . . occurs after you become aware of a particular thought by Listening In and using Underlining to decide that the thought is undesirable and needs to be stopped. The technique itself involves producing a word—"STOP"—in your internal thinking. Whenever the undesirable thought or thoughts occur, you give the command: STOP!

United States airlines do not permit smoking, but foreign carriers do.

When reserving a seat on an airline where smoking is permitted, make sure to ask for a seat as far from the smoking section as possible.

HOW TO APPLY STOPPING

In its straightforward way, Stopping is a high-powered technique for extinguishing your weakening thoughts or resolves. Whenever an undesirable message comes through, give the command: Stop. Try to block the thought as early as you can. Nip it in the bud. The forceful manner we described above will help. If possible, keep the thought from finishing itself. This will take some practice, but don't get discouraged. As you persevere, you'll become more adept at the technique, just as runners or swimmers or violinists do at the techniques they're trying to perfect.

Tough is the operative word here. If you've never been tough before, train yourself. Raise your voice. And when you give a command, make it a monologue. Don't let those weakening words or images of a cigarette have a chance. It's your show. It's your own mind. You are entitled to quash and rout invaders.

Here we come to a paradox. At the same time that you're being relentless with your negative thoughts, you want to be kind to yourself. Always keep in mind whose side you're on. You are not the enemy. The enemy is the negative desire for cigarettes. You don't want to add to your distress. Remember: You're on your side. Although you have to be harsh with the unpleasant thought, to Stop it, you don't extend the harshness to yourself.

Do not just Stop your damaging inner speech and leave yourself with an empty mind! Move on immediately to master:

SWITCHING

Switching deliberately interrupts damaging inner speech and replaces it with positive internal voices.

So far we've discussed the first three techniques of Inner Speech Therapy. You've learned to hear what's going on in your mind *(Listening In)*; to isolate the damaging messages *(Underlining);* and to stop them as soon as they begin *(Stopping)*. But what happens after you exorcise the demons? Minds don't stay empty. They fill up of their own accord, and that's precisely what you don't want yours to do. And unless you replace the damaging thought, it will return. That is a key point to remember.

Switching replaces bad thoughts with good ones. It can happen spontaneously, or it can be an intentional act on your part. Be sure to keep in mind that Switching can be intentional, that it can be learned. With a little diligence, you can train yourself to be good at it. Here are some tips on how to go about it.

First, remember that Stopping and Switching go hand in hand. As soon as you hear an undesirable thought, "I must have a cigarette," break in with the Stopping technique. Cut off the thought as early as you can and as many times as you have to. Some thoughts are doggedly persistent, but you can be more so.

The more quickly that Switching fills the void left by Stopping, the more effective it will be. Empty periods of mind time breed trouble. Try to be ready to fill any gaps with a Switching sentence you've prepared in advance. Think of something now and memorize it, so it will be available when you need it. Here are some examples of the kind of thing that works: "I'll switch to thinking about the promotion I got." Or "I'll switch to thinking about that day in the mountains. Next time I'm going to take the other trail, clear to the top." Be sure your Switching sentence is something that gives you pleasure or fortifies you in some way. The importance of what we think about has been understood since ancient times. In the words of the Bible, "Whatever is honorable . . . whatever is lovely . . . whatever is gracious . . . think about these things."

Have you ever been tired and down late in the day, and someone said, "Let's go out"? Your spirits picked up, and you began thinking about washing your face, putting on some fresh clothes, and hearing music in your head.

That is the experience of *Reorienting*. You reoriented the direction of your thinking. Your mood changed as you began to focus on a different target. The thing that produced your new enthusiasm was a reoriented thought. This is the power of Technique No. 5:

REORIENTING

Reorienting means to change the direction of your thinking. Your thinking deliberately focuses on a different target. If you are thinking of a cigarette, work on thinking about something completely different: a wonderful movie, or the compliment about your work you got from your boss. Change the direction of your thinking and you will change the direction you move today—and every day from now on. When you are in trouble, find a directing circumstance that positively demands your attention.

Switching and Reorienting have much in common, but there is an important difference. You will find it useful, when you are either anxious or fearful that you will never be able to quit smoking, to follow this fifth step of *Reorienting*.

Switching is an immediate thinking technique which should follow immediately after Stopping. Stopping alone is not enough, because your mind abhors a vacuum, and some thought will arrive momentarily and fill that vacuum if you do not deliberately choose a thought to occupy your mind. Your conscious choice of a useful thought will be far more helpful than letting an automatic thought take over.

The best Switching is toward an idea that begins to solve the immediate problem at hand. If that is not possible at the moment, then it is valuable for you to have some pleasant and successful thoughts memorized in advance to Switch into place. Eventually those affirming thoughts about yourself and your world can become your automatic thoughts. Many people, of course, do not believe that comforting thoughts can ever become automatic. You were not born with your thought patterns. You learned them. And if some of those habitual thoughts are not doing you much good, you can learn a different and more serviceable pattern of inner speech.

Reorienting, in contrast to Switching, is a much broader technique. You can Reorient to a grander view of your life. You can learn to see yourself differently. You can learn to see the world around you differently, in big and little ways.

Concentrate on an attractive goal and actively change the focus of your attention; you will feel much more in command, calmer, and more competent. You will understand that you have the will and ability to quit smoking.

Visualize yourself doing a job well. For example, people interested in sports learned that they could do better by watching successful rehearsals in their minds; they were able to hit a golf ball better, improve their skiing, and almost immediately cope with all sorts of physical activity that had previously frustrated them. They Reoriented from a clumsy, inept image of themselves to a smooth professional one, in which they were working calmly.

What follows is a wonderful example of relaxation therapy using Reorientation. This is accomplished by visualizing a relaxing blue-water rafting trip down a scenic canyon.

**Pack away all those ashtrays that are
placed on tables around the house.**

*If you must have a cigarette, you'll have to go to
the trouble of getting an ashtray from the draw-
er—and just remove one. Be sure to wash the
ashtray immediately after you smoke and put it
away again.*

THE GREAT CANYON TRIP

Often when patients ask Dr. Martorano how they
can relax when they're experiencing the irritability and
tension of withdrawal from cigarettes, he recommends
a mental trip via raft down a canyon.

Your mind is the key to relaxation. If you follow this
simple exercise, you can teach your body to relax.

First start by finding a quiet place where you can lie
down with a pillow under your head. After you lie
down, let yourself become aware of your breathing.
Measure each breath so that each breath is deeper and
slower than the one before.

Start counting backward in your mind from one
hundred. Count back slowly with each deep breath,
being careful to make each breath *deeper* and *slower*
than the one before. Instruct yourself to let your muscles relax and go limp with each deep breath.

Gradually you will find your body relaxing. Now let
your head go limp; your eyelids are getting heavier and
heavier and you begin to feel that you can't keep them
open.

As you do this, you will notice that it is getting harder and harder to count back as you continue breathing deeply and more slowly.

Now your body is limp and your eyes are closed.

Picture yourself on a large gray rubber raft, gently floating down a beautiful, slowly moving blue river at the bottom of a deep canyon. As you look up, you can see canyon walls on which are reflected deep purple shadows.

Now feel the water push at your body through the raft, gently massaging you. Let yourself relax as you imagine the raft lazily floating down the river, keeping your closed eyes fixed on the tiny bit of sky visible high above the canyon walls. Gradually your body will start to feel as if it's floating weightlessly. Keep counting backward as you continue to breathe deeply and slowly. Let your whole body breathe. The numbers are getting harder and harder to recall as you fall into a deeper state of relaxation.

Keep counting backward as the raft continues down the gentle canyon river, letting your body go limp. Enjoy the slow feeling of relaxation as you float down the river. Feel the warm sun shine down the canyon and gradually relax your body with warmth as you drift along.

Keep breathing more and more slowly. Your body will continue to unwind until your muscles are totally limp as you drift out of the canyon into a wide valley filled with warm sunlight. You are now totally relaxed and at peace with yourself.

YOU ARE IN CONTROL!

The Five-Step Plan has shown how you can be a stronger person. You can control those negative, destructive thoughts that kept you reaching for a cigarette. Never underestimate the importance of your mind and its ability to hold physical cravings at bay.

One former three-pack-a-day smoker said that he decided to quit when he realized he was not in control of his life.

"I couldn't stand the idea of being a slave. And that's how I thought of it—a slave to cigarettes. Once my mind was programmed to reject smoking, my body followed along."

This is the time to start taking charge of your thoughts; when you do that, your physiological needs will falter and slowly succumb.

Try not to flounder about—pushed and pulled by the dangerous desire for cigarettes. Understand that this much of your destiny is in your hands.

FOUR

PREPARING FOR CELLULAR NUTRITION

Micronutrients and phytochemicals do not require prescriptions and can be obtained at health food stores, as well as some pharmacies and supermarkets. Of course, before you embark on this or any other program, you should talk to your doctor.

After learning about micronutrients and phytochemicals, the next step is to learn how *much* of each you should take, and *when* you should take them. They work best when combined with macronutrients, or what we call Power Foods.

"What are Power Foods?" one cigarette smoker asked. "If I'm supposed to live on tofu and celery sticks you can forget it."

Not everyone can quit smoking cold turkey.

*To do it gradually, here's one way to make get-
ting at a cigarette a little harder. Wrap your
package of cigarettes neatly in gift paper and
secure it with a rubber band. Every time you
want a cigarette you have to go through the
trouble of unwrapping that package. And after
you take out one cigarette, make sure to wrap
the package again.*

MACRONUTRIENTS OR POWER FOODS

Power Foods are not the foods you love to hate, and
only eat because you think they're good for you or will
help you lose weight.

Power Foods are foods that you like and are familiar with. They are rich in protein and complex carbohydrates and provide your body with a steady stream
of glucose, which keeps your blood sugar levels from
dropping precipitously. When your blood sugar goes
down, you become hungry—usually for a chocolate
bar. But when your blood sugar stays at a steady level,
your appetite remains under control, and you feel
good.

In addition to keeping blood sugar on an even keel,
foods rich in protein and complex carbs contain vitamins, minerals, and fiber. Vitamins and minerals keep
you alert, and fiber helps decrease your appetite.

All those good things cannot be said for the *simple* carbohydrates—candy bars, ice cream, cake, white bread, cookies, pastas. That fat, sweet, and starchy stuff enters your bloodstream too fast. Your blood sugar hits a high, the food is quickly absorbed, and your blood sugar takes a precipitous drop. If you ever wonder why you're hungry half an hour after eating a candy bar, that's why. Besides, it's also a case of "a moment on the lips, a lifetime on the hips."

What are the Power Foods? Something exotic? Expensive? No, they are familiar foods that provide a continuous supply of fuel (glucose) to the brain without precipitating an overproduction of insulin that drives blood sugar down, causing a massive surge of appetite.

Here are the basic categories of Power Foods: meat, poultry, and fish. Vegetables and fruits. Whole-grain breads. Dairy foods. Nuts. To go into more detail, here's what to emphasize and what to minimize:

MEAT, POULTRY, FISH . . . You already know that lean is best. This means that it's a good idea to opt for chicken or fish over red meat, and to go for the leaner cuts when eating meat. It does not mean that you can never, ever eat a well-marbled steak again. It does mean that you should pay attention to those sensible thoughts that say, "Hey, you don't need a fat fix every day."

VEGETABLES . . . Hurray for the veggies! They're loaded with vitamins, minerals, fiber. And they can fill you up without filling you out.

There are some vegetables, however, that should be a sometimes thing: avocados—they contain fat; car-

rots—so crunchy, so sweet, so loaded with sugar; potatoes, beans, peas, corn, acorn squash—more starch
than you need every day.

FRUITS . . . What would we do without them?
They make such good desserts and wonderful snacks.
They're sweet and rich with vitamins and minerals and
fiber. Reach for fruit when you want a snack.

However, not all fruits are created equal: Bananas,
cherries, and pineapple should not be a daily treat
because they have a high sugar content.

BREADS . . . Go for the whole grains. Avoid the
soft white breads—hamburger buns and hot dog rolls
included. They contain little fiber and too much starch
and simple carbs. A good, chewy slice of rye or a
pumpernickel roll will do a lot to keep hunger pangs
away.

DAIRY FOODS . . . Some cheeses contain less fat
than others—naturally. And some cheeses have been
reinvented to contain less fat. We think that a small
slice of an interestingly flavored natural cheese will go
further toward satisfying than a large hunk of a manu-
factured low-fat cheese. But that decision is yours, as
is whether you should use whole, 2%, or 1% milk in
your coffee or on your cereal.

If a small amount of whole milk in your coffee will
keep hunger from your door—and you know that
hunger can lead to the need for a cigarette—go for it.
Life is a series of trade-offs. Have the whole milk and
substitute an apple for a wedge of cheese when it's
snack time.

NUTS . . . They can be a satisfying, protein-rich
snack. Should you eat nuts every day? No, but a small

amount of crunchy, chewy nuts can help you stay away from something far more fattening—like a chocolate bar.

"That's it?" you're saying. "But that's what I eat all the time." Right, but do you?

A lot of people talk that talk, but in truth not all walk that walk. For example: You eat a hamburger for lunch; that's meat, right? But if it's a fast-food hamburger, it's probably two ounces of meat—more fat than meat—and that sad little hamburger is sitting on a humongous hamburger bun. A bun so squishy and fiberless that you could press it together and turn it into an eraser. That thin hamburger—and that's the only thin thing about this meal—is not satisfying and far from filling, so you order a large bag of fries. Fiber there, sure, but mostly it's starch and lots of fat. With that you probably order a diet soda. Well, that's good, right? Wrong!

Aspartame, the sugar substitute used in most diet sodas, has been shown to provoke a lowering of blood sugar. You might not notice the effects of that drop immediately—that tired, and hungry feeling—because it takes about an hour and a half *after* you drink that soda for the effects to be felt.

A soft drink containing sugar is often cited as having "empty calories," but a diet soft drink could be called "empty noncalories." And according to some research, aspartame might prevent the exit of fat from your cells. If you're worried about weight, diet soda is probably not the way to go, nor is any severe form of dieting which encourages too much of a reduction in calories. This frequently backfires, because your body responds by slowing down your metabolism.

> ### Try to exercise at least
> ### fifteen minutes each day.
>
> *Walk, Exercycle in front of the TV, join a gym. Maybe you haven't realized it yet, but cigarettes have affected your physical stamina and ability to breathe. Smoking is not allowed in a gym, and it's a great place to reduce stress and rebuild your body, which may have been hurt by cigarettes. You can't smoke while on a treadmill, and no one puffs away at a cigarette while doing aerobics.*

GETTING READY TO QUIT

As you can see, quitting smoking calls for a double effort: You must get your mind into gear so that you truly believe that you can live without cigarettes, and you must get your body physically accustomed to doing without nicotine.

CONTINUE SMOKING

Knowing that, you can understand why you can't jump into the Cellular Nutrition Program. It takes advance planning. Take a look at your calendar. Circle a date three weeks ahead! That is *The Day*—the day you will stop smoking!

Meanwhile, continue smoking (we can't believe we said that, but we mean continue smoking *only* for the next three weeks) and move on to the first of four guides:

KEEPING TRACK

1. Buy a small notebook and make a note of the times that you eat—and what you eat—each day. This is an important habit to establish. When you start the Cellular Nutrition Program in three weeks, you will want to keep your blood sugar *level* so that you don't suffer those enervating appetite swings which keep you reaching for a candy bar.

EAT OFTEN!

2. Now that you know what times you eat, start the habit of never going more than two and half hours without eating a snack. No, don't panic, the snacks we recommend will not send your weight skyrocketing. Instead, your body will experience an even flow of blood sugar. This is crucially important because your brain will be fueled by two major substances—oxygen and glucose (sugar)—and you need to eat frequently to avoid a plummeting blood sugar. We can't repeat this often enough: Once your blood sugar drops precipitously, your brain starts signaling you to smoke or eat.

   It is especially important to eat right at bedtime so that you don't wake in the morning with your low blood sugar screaming at you to get up and get that first morning cigarette.

BUT, DON'T EAT . . .

3. Think about what you should *not* eat. Simple sugars and simple carbohydrates such as cakes, candy, and fruit juices are the worst culprits. Understanding why will strengthen your resolve to avoid them, so here goes:

When your blood sugar drops, you reach for a cigarette. But now that you're doing your best to avoid smoking rather than reaching for a cigarette, you reach for something sweet. This sends your blood sugar up really fast, and you feel good—but only for a short time as your insulin overreacts and drives your blood sugar back down. Paradoxically, your blood sugar often goes even lower than before the whole cycle started, and your brain starts screaming for *something:* "Give me a cigarette or give me a candy bar—and make it quick!"

That's why it's important to avoid foods with simple sugars! You know about candy, ice cream, cake, and soft drinks, but do you also know about alcohol and fruit juice?

Alcohol causes your blood sugar to rise so rapidly that it manages to bypass the liver and signals the brain directly to take in more sugar . . . *or smoke a cigarette.* The two things are synonymous. Even one glass of wine can cause blood sugar to drop for days because the alcohol blocks a delicate but important operation in your body called *glucogenesis*. Glucogenesis occurs when your blood sugar drops and your brain signals your body to send stored glucose into the bloodstream. But if glucogenesis is blocked, instead of using the stored glucose, you'll reach for food that will supply additional glucose—another reason for weight gain. If you're at a party, or invited for an after-work drink, ask for a glass of club soda with ice and a wedge of lime. Delicious and trendy, too.

The next substance that makes it hard to stop smoking will come as a big surprise . . . *citrus juice*. This is not the benign, healthy substance it is supposed to be . . . not when it's drunk by a susceptible person with low blood sugar. Citrus juice can cause your blood sugar to rise too rapidly and your brain to beg, getting your insulin to overreact and causing you to reach for a cigarette or a sweet.

You have to learn to cope with a "big lie" that has become endemic to our culture. Not all health foods are healthy. Particularly those that say they avoid sugar by using only *fruit juices*. Don't be fooled—all fruit juices, even freshly squeezed ones, are simple sugars, which have the same negative effect on your body as any other sugar. You need to read every label to make sure to avoid those as much as possible.

The same goes for all those other sugars: fructose, corn syrup, honey. If you want to quit smoking, you can't allow your blood sugar to be driven up. You won't be able to avoid every bit of sugar, but it's a good idea to start reading labels now. A loaf of packaged white bread, you might be surprised to discover, may contain fructose, corn syrup, and honey. Does this mean that you will never, ever be able to eat a slice of white bread again? No, it doesn't mean that—but once you know about those hidden sugars, you can cut down on foods that contain them. Perhaps you eat dry cereal for breakfast—no, no, you would never eat the sugar-frosted variety, but many of the "no-sugar-added" cereals are made with sugar and/or corn syrup. You know about cookies, but many crackers are prepared with sugar as well. Manufacturers of low-fat or no-fat cookies and cakes often compensate for the lack of fat by loading the products with sugar. Read labels!

ALMOST THERE

4. During the three weeks before you go on the Cellular Nutrition Program you will also start with some of the micronutrients.

Here's the schedule to follow:

Week One: Take one 40-milligram ginkgo biloba after breakfast.

Week Two: Take one 40-milligram ginkgo biloba after breakfast and another after dinner. Take one B vitamin after your midmorning snack.

Week Three: Continue with the ginkgo biloba, and the B vitamin, and add one 500-milligram lecithin with your bedtime snack.

You are now ready to start the Cellular Nutrition Program.

FIVE

GETTING WITH THE PROGRAM

It is now three weeks since you started preparing for the Cellular Nutrition Program. You woke this morning, and as usual, you reached for a cigarette. Or maybe you held off until you had that first cup or container of coffee in your hand.

But this is the first day of the rest of your wonderful, cigarette-free life. You won't need that cigarette to have energy and feel calm. Instead of the cigarette, you can have a satisfying breakfast: scrambled egg with Canadian bacon and rye toast.

We hear you saying, "I never eat that much food for breakfast."

Of course you don't. Instead of eating, you've been smoking. You've been starving your body, substituting nicotine for nutrients. But now you are going to eat . . . and eat! You'll combine meals you'll really enjoy with the micronutrients until cigarettes become not an ever-

present desire but a memory. And it won't take any-
where as long as you thought it might!

THE GOOD NEWS

Remember the diet gurus who used to scold when
it came to eating between meals? Well, on this program not only can you eat between meals, it's an
absolute must. Instead of three meals, you'll be eating six meals a day. There will be snacks between
breakfast and lunch, between lunch and dinner, and
before bedtime. True, those between-meal treats will
not be major food orgies, but they will keep you satisfied.

Must you eat between meals? Yes! You need those
small meals to keep your blood sugar from soaring up
or dropping down. Skip snack time and you may find
yourself raiding the refrigerator at 2:00 A.M. for that
pint of chocolate chip ice cream. But keep yourself
happily satisfied with foods containing protein and
complex carbohydrates and you'll be less likely to
reach for that chocolate-covered doughnut.

Remember when we told you to keep track of
the times you eat your meals? Take a look at your
notes. If you're like many dedicated smokers, your
notes might look like Daisy's before she embarked on
the Cellular Nutrition Program. Here's what she
wrote:

7:00 A.M.   I had one cup of black coffee—no sugar or cream.

9:30   I had another cup of coffee, black, at my desk with a cheese Danish—but the Danish was on the small side.

12:30 P.M. I went to lunch with my friends and ordered a hamburger, a small salad with lo-cal dressing, and a diet soda.

3:00   I drank a diet soda. (Some days I have iced tea.)

4:30   I knew I'd be working late, so I ate a chocolate bar and had some more black coffee.

8:30   When I got home I was too tired to cook the steak I had in the fridge, so I sent for take-out: Chinese—hot-and-sour soup and General Tzo's chicken, which I ate with brown rice and those great crispy fried noodles. My take-out place always sends along a diet soda and a sliced orange on the house, so I had those, too.

11:30   I got really hungry after watching "Seinfeld," so I ate a few spoonfuls of low-fat Häagen-Dazs—chocolate.

            I smoked about a pack and a half of cigarettes.

Does that sound like your day? And can't you just *hear* Daisy's entire body crying out for help?

Take a look at your own record of when and what you've been eating. Now turn the page! Or better still, buy a new notebook and start from the beginning.

Do you feel strained and tired from trying so hard not to smoke?

Drink a glass of water. As a matter of fact, drink many glasses of water. Just plain water? You bet! Water actually reduces the fatigue you may experience when you withdraw from nicotine. (Water also helps keep weight down, another plus.)

KEEPING RECORDS

It's important to keep a record of all your meals and the micronutrients you take with them. Without those records you might forget some micronutrients, and you will be more liable to skip a meal—or to eat simple sugars and carbohydrates. If you keep track of everything you eat, you'll be less likely to eat bad stuff.

Here's an example of how to create a daily chart listing all meals and micronutrients for each day:

Monday	Food	Micronutrients
BREAKFAST		
SNACK		
LUNCH		
SNACK		
DINNER		
SNACK		
Tuesday		
BREAKFAST		
SNACK		
LUNCH		
SNACK		
DINNER		
SNACK		
Wednesday		
BREAKFAST		
SNACK		
LUNCH		
SNACK		
DINNER		
SNACK		

Keep a record for each day, and leave space at the bottom of each day's page for the optional snack which you may have if you're having a late dinner.

Here are the foods you'll be enjoying on the Cellular Nutrition Program:

POWER BREAKFASTS

Fresh fruits: apples, pears, bananas, citrus fruits—but
    no citrus juices, not even the freshly squeezed ones.
    Berries, melons, peaches, plums, nectarines, kiwi.
    Pineapple, and cherries occasionally
Low-fat plain yogurt
Eggs
Cottage cheese as well as other cheeses
Canadian bacon
Protein leftovers from dinner the night before, such as
    roast or broiled meat, fish, chicken
Lean cold cuts
Whole-grain breads
Hot or cold sugar-free cereal
Milk for cereal
Green tea
Regular tea, coffee, herbal tea

POWER SNACKS

Sugar-free peanut butter
Whole-grain breads
Whole-grain crackers
Fresh fruit (see breakfast list)
Cottage cheese
Cheese
Rice cake
Soup
Raw vegetables: celery, bell peppers, fennel, cabbage,
    cucumber, lettuce, tomato

Green tea
Cappuccino
Lean cold cuts
Low-fat yogurt
Nuts

POWER LUNCHES

Salads, all kinds with vinaigrette or low-calorie dress-
    ing
Fish or shellfish: any kind, broiled, baked, grilled,
    steamed
Lean meats and fowl: chicken, turkey, rock cornish
    hen, beef, lamb, pork, veal (broiled, baked, grilled,
    roasted, steamed)
All vegetables except potatoes and beans
Sandwiches: cheese; lean meats, including cold cuts;
    fish or chicken salads, preferably from the spa side
    of the menu; lean hamburger. Sandwiches should be
    on whole-grain breads. Tea, coffee, herbal tea, green
    tea, club soda with wedges of lemon or lime
Soups

POWER DINNERS

Anything from the power lunches list; meats, fowl, and
    fish may also be braised, stewed, or sautéed.
All vegetables, and you may have potatoes, beans, or
    rice once a week.
All fruits, raw or cooked in a compote
Whole-grain breads

Now that you've read the food choices, we can hear you say, "But I never eat that much—especially not for breakfast." Of course you don't. And that's why, by the time you get to work or school, you're half-starved and you reach for a cigarette and a Danish.

The breakfasts on the program will keep you going until ten o'clock or maybe eleven, at which time you should have your first Power Snack. And the power snacks will keep you going until lunch.

And don't skip lunch—don't skip any meal or any snack. You'll get too hungry, your blood sugar will drop, and you'll reach for the usual dangerous combo: cigarettes and sweets.

Don't forget: Do not let more than two and a half hours pass between a meal and a snack. If you're working late, reach for a second snack *before* you head for home so you won't need a cigarette. This can be especially important if you're joining friends for a drink. You won't be so tempted by a bowl of chips or a dish of peanuts if you've kept your blood sugar level.

Does this mean that you can never, ever eat chips and salsa? The words *never, ever* are not part of the Stop Smoking, Stay Skinny Plan. What we are stressing is *moderation*. The only item that you will be giving up completely is an addictive, unhealthy, non-nutritional, potential killer—the cigarette.

You will not feel deprived if you follow the Menu Plan: If you don't feel like cooking, stop at a local salad bar for prepared veggies. Your local deli will be happy to send over salads with poached chicken or fish, or a rotisserie chicken. Chinese takeout is a possi-

bility when you order an assortment of wonderful
Asian vegetables with chicken, fish, or shellfish—the
trick here is to have these dishes steamed. Dessert can
be fresh fruit. At this stage avoid ice cream and
cakes—but this does not mean that once you get your
metabolism in synch, you will never be able to enjoy a
rich dessert.

THE LATE NIGHT SNACK

It's vital that you have a snack before you go to bed.
The longest period of time without food is between
dinner and breakfast. You wake up, your blood
sugar is really low, and you reach for a cigarette. But
if you eat a snack at bedtime, your blood sugar will
not drop precipitously during the night. Don't buy into the myth that if you eat at bedtime, you'll get fat.
The best way to keep from smoking—and overeat-
ing—is to make sure that you distribute fuel—food—
evenly to your brain throughout the day and the night.

One way to control your desire for a cigarette and
food is to have that nightly low-calorie snack. Do that
and you won't wake at 3:00 or 4:00 A.M. so ravenous
you'll rush to the fridge for that pint of chocolate ice
cream. And if that's not available, you'll dig into your
pocket for that package of M & M's left over from the
movies—or you'll reach for a cigarette.

How to avoid the need for after-midnight chocolate
or ice cream? Eat something that combines protein and
complex carbohydrates. This could be an apple or pear
with a small wedge of cheese, a slice of chicken or

turkey left over from dinner. You'll wake up feeling good, full of energy, not half-starved—and it will be easier to say no to that cigarette.

A WORD ABOUT PASTA

Pasta is delicious. It's also loaded with simple carbohydrates (starch)—the carbohydrate that can add weight. We've all read interviews in which famous Italian actresses and equally famous models say, "Sure I eat pasta—I eat everything."

How come they're so thin you ask? You're so careful about how much and what you eat. You starve yourself all day long and then scarf down a giant bowl of linguine with steamed broccoli rabe and red peppers for supper—and you don't understand why you can't keep your weight down, especially after you've given up smoking.

Maybe because a giant bowl of pasta is not such good stuff. A few pieces of ziti tossed with lots of fresh tomatoes and basil is fine, but a large helping of carb-loaded pasta? No way.

And those skinny stars who eat everything? Have a meal with them and you'll see a large quantity of veggies with just a few strands of angel hair peeking through. That's what *they* mean when they say they eat *everything*.

PORTION CONTROL

We don't specify amounts of food, because with three—and sometimes four—snacks each day, you won't want huge portions. The emphasis is on complex carbohydrates combined with a reasonable amount of protein. Eat enough to feel satisfied, but do not eat so much that you feel stuffed.

When does that fourth snack come into play? When more than two and half hours have passed after your afternoon snack and you're nowhere near having dinner. Choose any snack from the Power Snack list or from the Menu Plan. The raw vegetable snacks, which are crunchy, will give you the same sensation you get when eating potato chips or pretzels. They also are a great substitute for the oral satisfaction obtained from cigarettes.

READ LABELS

Just as you might have been fooled into thinking that a large quantity of pasta is a healthy meal, you may also have been fooled about simple sugars. Food labels can be deceptive. Jams and jellies, for example, may be labeled "sugar-free" because they are made with fruit juices. But those fruit juices have been distilled into a pure sugar syrup. Learn to read labels to be able to cut down on simple sugars, and stay away from foods with fructose, sucrose, corn syrup, and carob.

KEEPING WEIGHT DOWN BY EATING ENOUGH

Remember that you're working on giving up cigarettes, not on giving up food. We are not telling you to
overeat, but you should eat enough to keep your body
functioning at its energetic best. Three meals and three
snacks that combine protein and complex carbohydrates can keep your body in good shape, your brain
and appetite satisfied, your blood sugar on an even
keel. And remember that *not eating enough* can be just
as dangerous to your health as *eating too much.*
Anorexia is just as ugly as obesity.

AN IMPORTANT GUIDE

Remember to combine a small amount of protein—
meat, chicken, or fish—with a large amount of complex carbohydrates such as vegetables and fruits, and
take the micronutrients as directed.

COMBINING MEALS WITH MICRONUTRIENTS

We've told you about micronutrients, phytochemicals, macronutrients or Power Foods. Now, how do
you put it all together? Here's an example of one day's
timetable: Using the foods listed in the Power Foods
section, here's what you do:

With These Meals	*Take These Micronutrients*
Power Breakfast	one 40-milligram ginkgo biloba
Power Snack	one vitamin B complex one 200-milligram chromium picolinate
Power Lunch	one 500-milligram L-carnitine
Power Snack	one 30-milligram coenzyme 10
Power Dinner	one 40-milligram ginkgo biloba
Power Snack at Bedtime	one 500-milligram lecithin

We can't emphasize enough that there is nothing rigid about the Stop Smoking, Stay Skinny Program. Now that you know about the micronutrients, the phytochemicals, and the Power Foods, you can create your own daily menu. But if you want to take the easy way, follow our Thirty-Day Plan.

SIX

You Can Stop Smoking in Thirty Days!

Here's the Thirty-Day Plan that has everything: what to eat each day and which micronutrients to take with each meal. The phytochemicals will be in the foods, so you won't need supplements for them.

The menus offer many choices and we've provided recipes for all the starred dishes. Do you want to switch lunches and dinners around? That's fine. Would you rather substitute one dinner for another? That's okay, too. You won't have to eat two ounces of this or four ounces of that. Nor will you be forced to eat broccoli every Tuesday or salmon every Wednesday.

This is not a diet book—it's a multi-faceted program that combines foods that are high in complex carbohydrates and protein with the micronutrients that can mimic the effects of nicotine *without cigarettes*.

> **Put the money that you haven't used
> to buy a pack of cigarettes in a
> see-through container.**
>
> *Wow! Watch the money mount up!*

FAT, LOW FAT, NO FAT

As you've noticed in our list of Power Foods, we do not specify low-fat foods. We're sure you already know that the less fat you eat, the skinnier you'll be. However, we also feel that a small portion of the real stuff can be infinitely more satisfying than a larger portion of reduced-fat foods. And many low-fat foods, such as cheese or cake, compensate with added salt or sugar—not good for blood pressure or weight.

There are diet experts who advocate a high-fat diet, and that might seem enticing at first. But while those diets are rich in cream, butter, and well-marbled meat, they are low in the important and sustaining complex carbohydrates that can be found in fruits, vegetables, and whole grains.

When it comes to foods containing some fat, we believe in moderation—the middle way—as taught by the practitioners of the Chinese philosophy of Tao. And to bring that idea up to date, let's talk about the French—those chic people who cook with butter, eat foie gras, stay slim, and have fewer heart attacks than Americans.

It's called the French Paradox, but maybe it's not so paradoxical when you consider the smaller portions that they enjoy. And despite their well-deserved reputation for delicious pastries, the French don't indulge in simple sugars. They end meals with fresh fruit or a compote. Rich desserts are enjoyed at special fetes, or when Americans come visiting. The desserts in the recipe section are all based on fruit, and only a few recipes call for a small amount of sugar or honey.

We leave it to you to decide which cheeses to eat, and which milk to use in your coffee or on your cereal. It makes sense, though, when faced with a choice of a regular tuna, salmon, or chicken salad or a spa version of those salads, as they are now listed on many menus, to go for the spa salad. And why waste calories on high-fat cottage cheese when the pot-style low-fat cottage cheese tastes better? That's so easy, you might as well take advantage of the offer. Are lean meats better for you than fat-laden meats? Sure, but you already knew that.

The menus offer many choices, and in time, when your body stabilizes, you'll also be able to dip a spoon into a dish of chocolate ice cream.

The Menu Plan recommends which micronutrients to take with each meal. While these supplements have not as yet been FDA tested, that might change now that there is an office of Alternative Medicine in the National Institutes of Health. Before you start this or any other program, check with your doctor.

Indulge in one of those fancy bottled waters.

Instead of reaching for a cigarette, pour some of that nice bubbly stuff into a glass. If you're home, add a slice of lime or lemon.

LOOKING AHEAD

No program works for everyone, but we believe you will be able to throw away those cigarettes at the end of the month and still be happy when you look in the mirror!

SEVEN

THIRTY-DAY MENU PLAN*

DAY ONE	MICRONUTRIENTS
BREAKFAST Scrambled egg with Canadian bacon Rye toast Tea, coffee, or herbal tea	one 40-milligram ginkgo biloba
SNACK Banana	one vitamin B complex
LUNCH Salad of mixed vegetables with slices of turkey and vinaigrette dressing Club soda with a wedge of lemon or lime	one 200-milligram chromium picolinate one 500-milligram L-carnitine

*Recipes follow for all dishes containing asterisks.

DAY ONE	MICRONUTRIENTS
SNACK Rice cake with peanut butter	one 30-milligram coenzyme 10
SUPPER Chicken with Broccoli and Red Bell Pepper* Cucumber and onion salad Melon	one 40-milligram ginkgo biloba
BEDTIME SNACK Pear and cheese	one 500-milligram lecithin

DAY TWO	MICRONUTRIENTS
BREAKFAST	
Cereal with milk	one 40-milligram
Tea, coffee, or herbal tea	ginkgo biloba
SNACK	
Hearts of celery with cheese	one vitamin B complex
LUNCH	
Fisherman's Chowder*	one 200-milligram
Whole-grain bread	chromium picolinate
Tomato and onion salad	one 500-milligram
	L-carnitine
SNACK	
Feta cheese and whole-grain cracker	one 30-milligram coenzyme 10
SUPPER	
Broiled flank steak	one 40-milligram
Baked potato	ginkgo biloba
Sautéed mushrooms	
Honeydew melon	
BEDTIME SNACK	
Apple	one 500-milligram lecithin

Handwritten annotations: next to ginkgo biloba — "anti Oxydant / Circulation"; next to coenzyme 10 — "anti OXIDANT / Circulation"

DAY THREE	MICRONUTRIENTS

BREAKFAST
 	
Slices of leftover flank
   steak
Whole-grain bread
Tea, coffee, or herbal tea
	one 40-milligram
	   ginkgo biloba

SNACK Banana and green tea	one vitamin B complex

LUNCH
 	
Steamed asparagus with
   lemon
Broiled fillet of sole or
   flounder
Iced coffee
	one 200-milligram
	   chromium picolinate
	one 500-milligram
	   L-carnitine

SNACK Pear	one 30-milligram coenzyme 10

SUPPER
 	
Stir-fried Broccoli with
   Garlic and Tomatoes*
Lean hamburger on
   baguette
	one 40-milligram
	   ginkgo biloba

BEDTIME SNACK
 	
Peanut butter on rice
   cake
	one 500-milligram
	   lecithin

DAY FOUR	MICRONUTRIENTS
BREAKFAST Cottage cheese with fresh pineapple Tea, coffee, or herbal tea	one 40-milligram ginkgo biloba
SNACK Low-fat plain yogurt	one vitamin B complex
LUNCH Open-face turkey sandwich topped with tomato slices Iced tea	one 200-milligram chromium picolinate one 500-milligram L-carnitine
SNACK Cappuccino	one 30-milligram coenzyme 10
SUPPER Monkfish Steaks in Orange-Ginger Sauce* Steamed green beans Whole-grain bread Half grapefruit	one 40-milligram ginkgo biloba
BEDTIME SNACK Baked pear	one 500-milligram lecithin

DAY FIVE	MICRONUTRIENTS
BREAKFAST Poached egg with Canadian bacon Tea, coffee, or herbal tea	one 40-milligram ginkgo biloba
SNACK Chicken-vegetable soup and whole-grain crackers	one vitamin B complex
LUNCH Whole-wheat bagel with cheese slices and cucumber Club soda with wedge of lime	one 200-milligram chromium picolinate one 500-milligram L-carnitine
SNACK Low-fat plain yogurt	one 30-milligram coenzyme 10
SUPPER Chicken baked with Hot Peppers and Tomato* Steamed cauliflower Baked apple	one 40-milligram ginkgo biloba
BEDTIME SNACK Endive leaves spread with peanut butter	one 500-milligram lecithin

DAY SIX	MICRONUTRIENTS
BREAKFAST Cereal with milk and banana Tea, coffee, or herbal tea	one 40-milligram ginkgo biloba
SNACK Blueberries	one vitamin B complex
LUNCH Chicken broth Spinach and mushroom salad Whole-grain roll Tea	one 200-milligram chromium picolinate one 500-milligram L-carnitine
SNACK Hearts of celery	one 30-milligram coenzyme 10
SUPPER Stir-fried Cabbage with Cardamom* Roast loin of pork Sugar-free applesauce	one 40-milligram ginkgo biloba
BEDTIME SNACK Pear	one 500-milligram lecithin

DAY SEVEN	MICRONUTRIENTS
BREAKFAST Leftover roast loin of pork Cherry tomatoes Tea, coffee, or herbal tea	one 40-milligram ginkgo biloba
SNACK Grapefruit	one vitamin B complex
LUNCH Mixed green salad with tuna packed in water, drained Coffee or tea	one 200-milligram chromium picolinate one 500-milligram L-carnitine
SNACK Cheese slices with Nectarine Relish*	one 30-milligram coenzyme 10
SUPPER Stir-fried Chicken with Snow Peas* Braised Celery* Raspberries	one 40-milligram ginkgo biloba
BEDTIME SNACK Apple	one 500-milligram lecithin

DAY EIGHT	MICRONUTRIENTS
BREAKFAST Poached egg Whole-grain bread Tea, coffee, or herbal tea	one 40-milligram ginkgo biloba
SNACK Cup of chicken consommé	one vitamin B complex

LUNCH.
 	
Gazpacho with Scallops*
Whole-grain roll
Tea or coffee
	one 200-milligram
	  chromium picolinate
	one 500-milligram
	  L-carnitine

SNACK Hearts of celery	one 30-milligram coenzyme 10

SUPPER
 	
Steamed artichoke
Broiled chicken
Baked potato
Tomato and cucumber
  slices
	one 40-milligram
	  ginkgo biloba

BEDTIME SNACK Melon	one 500-milligram lecithin

DAY NINE	MICRONUTRIENTS
BREAKFAST Low-fat plain yogurt with fresh peach slices Tea, coffee, or herbal tea	one 40-milligram ginkgo biloba
SNACK Fresh orange slices	one vitamin B complex
LUNCH Sardine sandwich on whole-grain bread with sliced onion Green tea	one 200-milligram chromium picolinate one 500-milligram L-carnitine
SNACK Minestrone soup	one 30-milligram coenzyme 10
SUPPER Fennel, endive, and orange salad Cabbage Rolls* Cantaloupe	one 40-milligram ginkgo biloba
BEDTIME SNACK Hearts of celery	one 500-milligram lecithin

DAY TEN	MICRONUTRIENTS
BREAKFAST Tangerine Farmer's cheese Whole-grain roll Coffee, tea, or herbal tea	one 40-milligram ginkgo biloba

SNACK
 	
Florets of cauliflower
    with Raita Dip*
	one vitamin B
	    complex

LUNCH
 	
Pear-Ginger Salad*
Club soda with lemon
    wedge
	one 200-milligram
	    chromium picolinate
	one 500-milligram
	    L-carnitine

SNACK Nectarine	one 30-milligram coenzyme 10
SUPPER Roast leg of lamb Wild rice Steamed zucchini Apple	one 40-milligram ginkgo biloba

BEDTIME SNACK
 	
Peanut butter on whole-
    grain cracker
	one 500-milligram
	    lecithin

DAY ELEVEN	MICRONUTRIENTS
BREAKFAST Omelette made with left-over zucchini Tea, coffee, or herbal tea	one 40-milligram ginkgo biloba
SNACK Grapefruit	one vitamin B complex

LUNCH
 	
Beef broth
Assorted roasted vegetables
Banana
Tea or coffee
	one 200-milligram
	   chromium picolinate
	one 500-milligram
	   L-carnitine

SNACK Cheese slice on whole-grain cracker	one 30-milligram coenzyme 10
SUPPER Chinese takeout: Steamed assorted vegetables Steamed Shrimp or prawns with broccoli and baby corn Orange slices	one 40-milligram ginkgo biloba
BEDTIME SNACK Vanilla-flavored Fruit Compote*	one 500-milligram lecithin

DAY TWELVE	MICRONUTRIENTS
BREAKFAST	
Cereal with milk and strawberries Tea, coffee, or herbal tea	one 40-milligram ginkgo biloba
SNACK	
Cucumber sticks	one vitamin B complex
LUNCH	
Open-face roast beef sandwich on whole-wheat baguette Green salad Club soda	one 200-milligram chromium picolinate one 500-milligram L-carnitine
SNACK	
Cottage cheese	one 30-milligram coenzyme 10
SUPPER	
Eggplant and Ginger Appetizer* Poached salmon Steamed green peas Vanilla-flavored Fruit Compote	one 40-milligram ginkgo biloba
BEDTIME SNACK	
Peanut butter on cracker	one 500-milligram lecithin

DAY THIRTEEN	MICRONUTRIENTS
BREAKFAST Egg scrambled with green pepper Tea, coffee, or herbal tea	one 40-milligram ginkgo biloba
SNACK Whole-grain cracker with peanut butter	one vitamin B complex
LUNCH Steamed shrimp over snow peas, broccoli, and water chestnuts Tea	one 200-milligram chromium picolinate one 500-milligram L-carnitine
SNACK Grape and Cheese Salad*	one 30-milligram coenzyme 10
SUPPER Curried Chicken in Yogurt Sauce with Peanuts* Basmati rice Cantaloupe	one 40-milligram ginkgo biloba
BEDTIME SNACK Half pumpernickel bagel with cottage cheese	one 500-milligram lecithin

DAY FOURTEEN	MICRONUTRIENTS
BREAKFAST Grapefruit Half pumpernickel bagel Poached egg Tea, coffee, herbal tea	one 40-milligram ginkgo biloba
SNACK Beef broth	one vitamin B complex
LUNCH Fresh fruit salad in half cantaloupe	one 200-milligram chromium picolinate one 500-milligram L-carnitine
SNACK Sliced turkey Whole-grain roll	one 30-milligram coenzyme 10
SUPPER Carrot-Ginger Soup* Boned shad, broiled with lemon wedges Mixed green salad Low-fat frozen yogurt	one 40-milligram ginkgo biloba
BEDTIME SNACK Pear	one 500-milligram lecithin

DAY FIFTEEN	MICRONUTRIENTS

BREAKFAST
 	
Cereal with milk and
    blueberries
Tea, coffee, or herbal tea
	one 40-milligram
	    ginkgo biloba

SNACK Salt-free cashew nuts	one vitamin B complex

LUNCH
 	
Mixed green salad
Boiled ham
Whole-grain roll
Tea or coffee
	one 200-milligram
	    chromium picolinate
	one 500-milligram
	    L-carnitine

SNACK Banana	one 30-milligram coenzyme 10

SUPPER
 	
Asparagus vinaigrette
Lamb, Zucchini, and
    Mushroom Kebabs*
Pineapple Fruit Salad
    with Ginger-Lime
    Dressing*
	one 40-milligram
	    ginkgo biloba

BEDTIME SNACK Apple	one 500-milligram lecithin

DAY SIXTEEN	MICRONUTRIENTS

BREAKFAST
 	
Cottage cheese with
    leftover pineapple fruit
    salad
Tea, coffee, or herbal tea
	one 40-milligram
	    ginkgo biloba

SNACK Celery hearts	one vitamin B complex

LUNCH
 	
Roast chicken
Grilled tomatoes
Grilled mushrooms
Tea or coffee
	one 200-milligram
	    chromium picolinate
	one 500-milligram
	    L-carnitine

SNACK Cheese Whole-grain roll	one 30-milligram coenzyme 10

SUPPER
 	
Baked Salmon and Celery
    Casserole*
Lentil salad
Vanilla-flavored Fruit
    Compote*
	one 40-milligram
	    ginkgo biloba

BEDTIME SNACK Peanut butter on rice cake	one 500-milligram lecithin

DAY SEVENTEEN	MICRONUTRIENTS
BREAKFAST Cheese slice on whole wheat bread, broiled Tea, coffee, or herbal tea	one 40-milligram ginkgo biloba
SNACK Apricot	one vitamin B complex
LUNCH Tomato stuffed with salmon salad Semolina bread Iced tea	one 200-milligram chromium picolinate one 500-milligram L-carnitine
SNACK Chicken gumbo soup	one 30-milligram coenzyme 10
SUPPER Carrot Salad* Broiled chicken Boiled red-jacket potato Steamed broccoli Nectarine	one 40-milligram ginkgo biloba
BEDTIME SNACK Banana	one 500-milligram lecithin

DAY EIGHTEEN	MICRONUTRIENTS

BREAKFAST
 	
Scrambled egg with
  Canadian bacon
Tea, coffee, or herbal tea
	one 40-milligram
	  ginkgo biloba

SNACK Grapefruit	one vitamin B complex

LUNCH
 	
Lentil soup
Mixed vegetable salad
Club soda with wedge of
  lime
	one 200-milligram
	  chromium picolinate
	one 500-milligram
	  L-carnitine

SNACK Strawberries	one 30-milligram coenzyme 10

SUPPER
 	
Pork with Ginger and
  Vegetables*
Sugar-free applesauce
Whole wheat baguette
Orange
	one 40-milligram
	  ginkgo biloba

BEDTIME SNACK
 	
Cottage cheese with
  whole-grain cracker
	one 500-milligram
	  lecithin

DAY NINETEEN	MICRONUTRIENTS
BREAKFAST Toasted oat bran English muffin Poached egg Tea, coffee, or herbal tea	one 40-milligram ginkgo biloba
SNACK Celery hearts	one vitamin B complex
LUNCH Broiled steak Tomato and onion salad Whole-grain roll Coffee	one 200-milligram chromium picolinate one 500-milligram L-carnitine
SNACK Vegetable soup	one 30-milligram coenzyme 10
SUPPER Arugula, endive, and radicchio salad Shrimp and Scallop Cassoulet* Raspberries	one 40-milligram ginkgo biloba
BEDTIME SNACK Salt-free almonds	one 500-milligram lecithin

DAY TWENTY	MICRONUTRIENTS
BREAKFAST Cottage cheese with sliced pear Tea, coffee, or herbal tea	one 40-milligram ginkgo biloba
SNACK Sliced fresh fennel	one vitamin B complex
LUNCH Broiled lean hamburger on whole-grain baguette with sliced onion Green salad Coffee or tea	one 200-milligram chromium picolinate one 500-milligram L-carnitine
SNACK Orange	one 30-milligram coenzyme 10
SUPPER Stuffed Fish Fillets with Ginger Sauce* Steamed green beans Blueberries	one 40-milligram ginkgo biloba
BEDTIME SNACK Peach	one 500-milligram lecithin

DAY TWENTY-ONE	MICRONUTRIENTS

BREAKFAST
Low-fat plain yogurt with
   fresh strawberries
Tea, coffee, or herbal tea
	one 40-milligram
	   ginkgo biloba

SNACK Cauliflower florets	one vitamin B complex

LUNCH
Sliced turkey
Whole-grain bread
Lettuce and tomato salad
Tea
	one 200-milligram
	   chromium picolinate
	one 500-milligram
	   L-carnitine

SNACK Apple	one 30-milligram coenzyme 10

SUPPER
Chicken consommé
Curried Lamb and Bas-
   mati Rice*
Tangerine
	one 40-milligram
	   ginkgo biloba

BEDTIME SNACK Feta cheese with pear	one 500-milligram lecithin

DAY TWENTY-TWO	MICRONUTRIENTS
BREAKFAST	
Cereal with milk and fresh raspberries	one 40-milligram ginkgo biloba
SNACK	
Hard-cooked egg	one vitamin B complex
LUNCH	
Roasted Red Peppers and Shrimp* Iced tea	one 200-milligram chromium picolinate one 500-milligram L-carnitine
SNACK	
Peanut butter on whole grain bread	one 30-milligram coenzyme 10
SUPPER	
Roast chicken Broiled tomato Stir-fried spinach Watermelon	one 40-milligram ginkgo biloba
BEDTIME SNACK	
Cheese with whole-grain cracker	one 500-milligram lecithin

DAY TWENTY-THREE	MICRONUTRIENTS
BREAKFAST Turkey slices Whole-grain bread, toasted Cucumber slices Tea, coffee, or herbal tea	one 40-milligram ginkgo biloba
SNACK Banana	one vitamin B complex
LUNCH French-Style Tuna Salad* Whole-grain baguette Tea or coffee	one 200-milligram chromium picolinate one 500-milligram L-carnitine
SNACK Salt-free pistachio nuts	one 30-milligram coenzyme 10
SUPPER Roast beef Baked potato Tomato and onion salad with basil Grapefruit	one 40-milligram ginkgo biloba
BEDTIME SNACK Apple	one 500-milligram lecithin

DAY TWENTY-FOUR	MICRONUTRIENTS
BREAKFAST Melon Leftover roast beef Whole-grain bread Tea, coffee, or herbal tea	one 40-milligram ginkgo biloba
SNACK Pear	one vitamin B complex

LUNCH
 	
Bean soup
Assorted grilled veg-
   etables
Mini whole wheat pita
   bread
Club soda with splash of
   cranberry juice
	one 200-milligram
	   chromium picolinate
	one 500-milligram
	   L-carnitine

SNACK Hearts of celery	one 30-milligram coenzyme 10
SUPPER Broiled shrimp Wild rice Sesame Green Beans* Cherries	one 40-milligram ginkgo biloba
BEDTIME SNACK Walnuts and sliced apple	one 500-milligram lecithin

DAY TWENTY-FIVE	**MICRONUTRIENTS**
BREAKFAST Cereal with milk Tea, coffee, or herbal tea	one 40-milligram ginkgo biloba
SNACK Cheese on whole-grain cracker	one vitamin B complex
LUNCH Tomato stuffed with spa- style chicken salad Whole-grain roll Green tea	one 200-milligram chromium picolinate one 500-milligram L-carnitine
SNACK Banana	one 30-milligram coenzyme 10
SUPPER Quick Mushroom Soup* Broiled Red Snapper Steamed green beans Cucumber, onion, and dill salad Melon	one 40-milligram ginkgo biloba
BEDTIME SNACK Apple	one 500-milligram lecithin

DAY TWENTY-SIX	MICRONUTRIENTS
BREAKFAST	
Egg scrambled with green onion Toasted whole-grain bread Tea, coffee, or herbal tea	one 40-milligram ginkgo biloba
SNACK	
Bell pepper slices	one vitamin B complex
LUNCH	
Chicken noodle soup Turkey Lettuce Wraps* Tea	one 200-milligram chromium picolinate one 500-milligram L-carnitine
SNACK	
Plum	one 30-milligram coenzyme 10
SUPPER	
Grapefruit Broiled Scallops Green beans and tomato sauté Raspberries	one 40-milligram ginkgo biloba
BEDTIME SNACK	
Farmer's cheese on whole-grain cracker	one 500-milligram lecithin

DAY TWENTY-SEVEN	MICRONUTRIENTS
BREAKFAST Rye bagel Cottage cheese Tea, coffee, or herbal tea	one 40-milligram ginkgo biloba
SNACK Orange	one vitamin B complex

LUNCH
 	
Broiled lamb chop with
    sliced tomatoes and
    peppers
Coffee
	one 200-milligram
	    chromium picolinate
	one 500-milligram
	    L-carnitine

SNACK
 	
Rice cake with peanut
    butter
	one 30-milligram
	    coenzyme 10

SUPPER
 	
Minestrone soup
Smoked Breast of
    Chicken and Bean
    Salad*
Semolina bread
Fresh pineapple
	one 40-milligram
	    ginkgo biloba

BEDTIME SNACK Blueberries	one 500-milligram lecithin

DAY TWENTY-EIGHT	MICRONUTRIENTS
BREAKFAST Cereal with milk Tea, coffee, or herbal tea	one 40-milligram ginkgo biloba
SNACK Cottage cheese with whole-grain cracker	one vitamin B complex

LUNCH
 	
Poached salmon
Mixed green salad
Iced tea
	one 200-milligram
	  chromium picolinate
	one 500-milligram
	  L-carnitine

SNACK Plain, low-fat yogurt	one 30-milligram coenzyme 10

SUPPER
 	
Black bean soup
Ginger Chicken with
  Lemon*
Fresh fruit cup
	one 40-milligram
	  ginkgo biloba

BEDTIME SNACK Banana	one 500-milligram lecithin

DAY TWENTY-NINE	MICRONUTRIENTS
BREAKFAST Mushroom omelette Toasted whole-grain bread Tea, coffee, or herbal tea	one 40-milligram ginkgo biloba
SNACK Sliced fresh fennel	one vitamin B complex
LUNCH Tomato soup Mini whole wheat pita stuffed with cheese and assorted raw vegetables Club soda with a splash of sugar-free grapefruit juice	one 200-milligram chromium picolinate one 500-milligram L-carnitine
SNACK Apple	one 30-milligram coenzyme 10
SUPPER Broiled steak Steamed spinach Baked potato Melon	one 40-milligram ginkgo biloba
BEDTIME SNACK Rice cake with farmer's cheese	one 500-milligram lecithin

DAY THIRTY	MICRONUTRIENTS
BREAKFAST Cereal with milk Tea, coffee, or herbal tea	one 40-milligram ginkgo biloba
SNACK Cheese with whole-grain cracker	one vitamin B complex
LUNCH Broiled swordfish steak Boiled red-jacket potato Mixed green salad Tea	one 200-milligram chromium picolinate one 500-milligram L-carnitine
SNACK Strawberries	one 30-milligram coenzyme 10
SUPPER Eggplant and Ginger Appetizer* Roast shoulder of veal Broiled Portobello mushrooms Mixed berry cup	one 40-milligram ginkgo biloba
BEDTIME SNACK Apple	one 500-milligram lecithin

EIGHT

RECIPES FOR THE CELLULAR NUTRITION PROGRAM

The recipes for the Program are easy, and the results are delicious. To prepare many of them, you'll have to stock up on two phytochemicals: *ginger* and *garlic*. One or both are used in many recipes, as is seasoned rice wine vinegar, which is mild and palatable even when used without oil. Where oil is called for, we prefer olive oil, which tastes good and, according to research, is best for your health. A small amount of fruit juice, and a very small amount of honey or sugar, can be found in a few recipes—but the amounts are so small they won't seriously affect the Cellular Nutrition Program.

STIR-FRIED BROCCOLI WITH GARLIC AND TOMATOES

1 pound broccoli florets
2 teaspoons olive oil
2 garlic cloves, pressed
Salt and freshly ground pepper to taste
2 plum tomatoes, chopped

1. Bring a large pot of water to boil and add broccoli. Blanch broccoli for three minutes. Drain.
2. Heat oil in a large, non-stick skillet. Add garlic and saute for one minute, stirring.
3. Add broccoli and stir-fry until broccoli is just tender. Season.
4. Transfer broccoli to a serving platter and garnish with chopped tomatoes.

SERVES: 4

COMFORT FOOD: CABBAGE ROLLS

1 medium head of cabbage
1 pound lean ground beef
1 large onion, grated
2 cloves garlic, pressed
2 tablespoons chopped flat or Italian parsley
1 egg, beaten
4 slices whole-grain bread
Salt and freshly ground pepper to taste
2 cups tomato sauce
1 cup vegetable, chicken, or beef broth
¼ teaspoon red pepper flakes (or to taste)

1. Parboil cabbage for ten to fifteen minutes in boiling water, until cabbage is barely tender. Drain and allow to cool.
2. In a bowl, combine beef, onion, garlic, parsley, and egg.
3. Soak bread briefly in warm water until just softened. Squeeze out excess water and add bread to meat mixture. Season and mix until ingredients are thoroughly combined.

4. Separate cabbage into individual leaves.
5. Spoon a small amount of meat mixture onto each leaf and roll, tucking in ends as you roll.
6. Combine tomato sauce and broth in a Dutch oven. Add pepper flakes and bring sauce to a simmer.
7. Carefully place cabbage rolls in Dutch oven.
8. Cover and simmer over low heat for one hour, or until cabbage is tender. Taste sauce and correct seasoning.

SERVES: 4–6

STIR-FRIED CABBAGE WITH CARDAMOM

2 teaspoons olive oil
1 small head cabbage, coarsely shredded
2 teaspoons light soy sauce
1 teaspoon ground cardamom
¼ teaspoon hot paprika (or to taste)
Salt to taste

1. Heat oil in a large, nonstick skillet.
2. Add cabbage and cook, stirring, for two minutes.
3. Add all remaining ingredients and continue cooking over medium-high heat, stirring occasionally,
   until cabbage is just tender.

SERVES: 4

CARROT-GINGER SOUP

1-pound package baby carrots
4 tablespoons grated fresh ginger
4 cups chicken broth
½ teaspoon ground cardamom
1 cup orange juice
Salt and freshly ground pepper to taste

1. Combine carrots, ginger, chicken broth, and cardamom in a soup pot.
2. Cook over low heat until carrots are very tender.
3. Puree soup in a food processor until smooth.
4. Return soup to pot and add orange juice. Bring soup to a simmer and season to taste.

SERVES: 4–6

CARROT SALAD

½ *pound baby carrots*
2 *garlic cloves*
½-*inch piece fresh ginger*
2 *teaspoons olive oil*
2 *teaspoons seasoned rice wine vinegar*

1. Using a food processor, grate carrots, garlic, and ginger, and transfer to a bowl.
2. Combine oil and vinegar and mix thoroughly. Spoon over carrot mixture and stir to combine.
3. Chill before serving.

SERVES: 4

BRAISED CELERY

2 teaspoons olive oil
2 garlic cloves, pressed
1 bunch celery, separated into stalks, trimmed,
   cut in half
2 cups chicken broth
½ cup dry white wine
Salt and freshly ground pepper to taste
1 tablespoon chopped flat or Italian parsley

1. Heat oil in a saucepan. Add garlic and saute over low heat for one minute.
2. Add celery, broth, and wine.
3. Cover and cook until celery is tender.
4. Season and garnish with parsley.

SERVES: 4

CHICKEN BAKED WITH HOT PEPPERS AND TOMATOES

2 teaspoons olive oil
1 2½-pound chicken, cut into 8 pieces
Salt and freshly ground pepper to taste
2 cups chicken broth
2 hot cherry peppers, cored, seeded, cut into strips
3 tomatoes, quartered

1. Preheat oven to 350 degrees.
2. Heat oil in a large, nonstick skillet. Add chicken and cook over medium-high heat until chicken is lightly browned on all sides.
3. Transfer chicken to an ovenproof casserole and season with salt and pepper.
4. Deglaze skillet by adding broth to skillet and cooking over high heat until liquid has reduced and is syrupy. Pour liquid over chicken.
5. Place hot pepper strips and tomato quarters around chicken.
6. Cover and bake until chicken is cooked through, from thirty to forty-five minutes.

SERVES: 4

SMOKED BREAST OF CHICKEN AND BEAN SALAD

½ pound green beans, cooked until just tender
1 cup cooked white beans
2 tablespoons olive oil
1 tablespoon balsamic vinegar
½ teaspoon Dijon mustard
1 garlic clove, pressed
1 pound smoked breast of chicken, cubed
Salt and freshly ground pepper to taste
1 small head of Romaine lettuce, chopped

1. Combine green beans and white beans in a bowl.
2. Combine oil, vinegar, mustard, and garlic. Mix thoroughly and spoon over beans.
3. Add chicken to beans and toss to combine. Season to taste.
4. Place chopped lettuce on a platter and top with bean-chicken mixture.

SERVES: 4–6

CHICKEN WITH BROCCOLI
AND RED BELL PEPPER

1 pound broccoli florets
2 teaspoons olive oil
1 red bell pepper, thinly sliced
2 skinless, boneless chicken breasts, cubed
1 cup chicken broth
4 green onions, thinly sliced
1 tablespoon chopped cilantro
2 tablespoons seasoned rice wine vinegar
1 tablespoon light soy sauce
Salt and freshly ground pepper to taste

1. Bring a large pot of water to boil and add broccoli. Blanch broccoli for three minutes. Drain.
2. Heat oil in a large, nonstick skillet. Add broccoli and red bell pepper. Cook, stirring for two minutes.
3. Add chicken and cook, stirring, one additional minute.
4. Add broth and continue cooking until chicken is cooked through, from ten to fifteen minutes.
5. Add green onions, cilantro, vinegar, and soy sauce. Continue cooking over medium high heat, stirring occasionally, for two minutes. Season to taste.

SERVES: 4

GINGER CHICKEN WITH LEMON

2 tablespoons grated fresh ginger
2 garlic cloves, pressed
4 tablespoons seasoned rice wine vinegar
1 tablespoon sesame oil
Juice of one large lemon
2 skinless and boneless chicken breasts, cut into large
   chunks
2 medium onions, quartered
2 red bell peppers, cut into 8 strips
8 large mushroom caps

1. Combine ginger, garlic, vinegar, oil, and lemon juice in a large bowl. Mix thoroughly.
2. Add chicken to bowl, toss, and refrigerate. Allow chicken to marinate for thirty minutes to an hour, turning once or twice in marinade.
3. Preheat oven to broil.
4. Thread chicken and vegetables on four skewers.
5. Place skewers on a broiling pan and spoon marinade over all.
6. Turn skewers once or twice and broil until chicken is lightly browned and cooked through, about ten to fifteen minutes.

SERVES: 4

STIR-FRIED CHICKEN WITH SNOW PEAS

2 teaspoons olive oil
½ pound snow peas
2 shallots, finely chopped
1 cup chicken broth
2 boneless and skinless chicken breasts, cut into strips
1 tablespoon balsamic vinegar
2 tablespoons light soy sauce
1 teaspoon hot pepper sauce (optional)

1. Heat oil in a large, nonstick skillet.
2. Add snow peas and shallots, and cook, stirring, for two minutes.
3. Add broth and chicken and cook, stirring, for two minutes.
4. Add all remaining ingredients. Stir to combine.
5. Cook over medium-high heat, stirring, until chicken is cooked through.

SERVES: 4

CURRIED CHICKEN IN YOGURT SAUCE WITH PEANUTS

2 teaspoons olive oil
4 garlic cloves, pressed
½ cup chicken broth
2 skinless, boneless chicken breasts, cubed
2 teaspoons curry powder
1 cup low-fat plain yogurt
¼ cup shelled peanuts

1. Heat oil in a large, nonstick skillet. Add garlic and sauté for one minute.
2. Add broth and chicken. Continue cooking, stirring occasionally, until chicken is cooked through.
3. While chicken cooks, combine curry powder and yogurt in a small bowl. Mix thoroughly.
4. Add curry-yogurt sauce to chicken. Cover and cook until all ingredients are heated through.
5. Transfer to a serving platter and garnish with peanuts.

SERVES: 4

EGGPLANT AND GINGER APPETIZER

2 teaspoons olive oil
4 small Italian or Japanese eggplant, peeled, each cut
*   lengthwise into 4 slices*
2 garlic cloves, minced
2 tablespoons grated fresh ginger
½ teaspoon hot pepper sauce
2 tablespoons light soy sauce
1 tablespoon seasoned rice wine vinegar

1. Heat oil in a large, nonstick skillet
2. Add eggplant, garlic, ginger, and hot pepper sauce. Cover and cook, turning eggplant occasionally, until eggplant is tender.
3. Add soy sauce and vinegar and continue cooking until liquid is absorbed.
4. Serve room temperature or chilled.

SERVES: 4

STUFFED FISH FILLETS
WITH GINGER SAUCE

4 sole or flounder fillets
1 stalk celery, finely chopped
2 shallots, minced
2 garlic cloves, pressed
1 teaspoon hot pepper sauce
Salt and freshly ground pepper to taste
2 teaspoons olive oil
2 green onions, finely chopped
3 tablespoons grated fresh ginger
1 cup dry white wine
Lemon wedges

1. Place fish fillets on a board or platter.
2. Combine celery, shallots, garlic, hot pepper sauce, and seasonings. Mix thoroughly.
3. Spoon one quarter of mixture in center of each fish fillet. Roll fish fillets carefully and reserve.
4. Heat oil in a large nonstick skillet.
5. Add green onion and ginger, and sauté, stirring, for one minute.
6. Place fish fillets, seam side down, in skillet.

7. Add wine. Cover and cook over low heat for about ten minutes, or until fish is cooked through.
8. Place fish fillets on a serving platter. Spoon liquid from skillet over fish and garnish with lemon wedges.

SERVES: 4

FISHERMAN'S CHOWDER

2 teaspoons olive oil
1 large onion, sliced
2 garlic cloves, pressed
6 very ripe tomatoes, chopped
1 red bell pepper, chopped
¼ teaspoon thyme
¼ teaspoon red pepper flakes
6 cups vegetable broth, or 3 cups vegetable broth and 3
    cups chicken broth
2 pounds fish fillets (cod, halibut, scrod, red snapper, or
    a combination)
Salt and freshly ground pepper to taste

1. Heat oil in a soup pot or Dutch oven. Add onion and
   garlic. Cook, stirring, for two minutes.
2. Add all remaining ingredients except for fish, salt,
   and pepper. Cover and cook over low heat for twenty minutes.
3. Cut fish into large pieces and add to pot.
4. Cover and cook for five to ten minutes or until fish
   is just cooked.
5. Season to taste.

SERVES: 4–6

VANILLA-FLAVORED FRUIT COMPOTE

1 pound very ripe peaches, pitted, cut into chunks
1 pound very ripe nectarines, pitted, cut into chunks
1 pound very ripe plums (any kind), pitted, cut into
  chunks
½ pound cherries
½ cup water
½ teaspoon vanilla extract
1 tablespoón sugar (or to taste)
Mint leaves for garnish (optional)

1. Combine fruit, water, and vanilla in a large pot.
2. Cover and bring to a simmer.
3. Taste liquid after fifteen minutes and add sugar.
4. Continue cooking until fruit is just tender.
5. Serve warm or chilled and garnish with mint leaves.

SERVES: 6

GAZPACHO WITH SCALLOPS

4 ripe tomatoes, coarsely chopped
1 small cucumber, peeled, chopped
1 medium onion, quartered
1 bell pepper, quartered
2 garlic cloves
1½ cups tomato juice
1 tablespoon balsamic vinegar
1 tablespoon olive oil
Dash of cayenne pepper
Salt and freshly ground pepper to taste
¾ pound sea scallops, cut in half, cooked

1. Combine all ingredients, except for scallops, in a food processor or blender and process until smooth.
2. Refrigerate until chilled.
3. To serve, ladle into soup bowls and top with scallops.

SERVES: 4–6

GINGER-LIME DRESSING

¼ cup honey
¼ cup orange juice
2 tablespoons lime juice
1 tablespoon grated fresh ginger
1 teaspoon grated lime peel

Combine all ingredients in a bowl. Mix well.

YIELD: ABOUT 1 CUP

GRAPE AND CHEESE SALAD
HOLLYWOOD STYLE

1 cup seedless green grapes, cut in half
1 cup seedless red grapes, cut in half
1 cup Bibb lettuce, coarsely chopped
3 tablespoons crumbled feta cheese
1 tablespoon seasoned rice wine vinegar

1. Combine grapes and mix well.
2. Place lettuce on a serving platter and top with grapes.
3. Sprinkle cheese over grapes.
4. Drizzle vinegar over all.

SERVES: 4

SESAME GREEN BEANS

1 pound green beans
Salt to taste
2 tablespoons tahini paste
Salt and freshly ground pepper to taste
1 tablespoon sesame seeds

1. Cut the tips off the beans and remove strings.
2. Bring enough water to a boil to cover beans. Add salt to taste.
3. Add beans to water and cook until beans are just tender.
4. Transfer beans to a colander, and let cold water run over beans to stop cooking. Drain beans thoroughly and transfer to a shallow serving dish.
5. Spoon tahini sauce over beans and toss. Season to taste.
6. Add sesame seeds and toss again. Chill before serving.

SERVES: 4

CURRIED LAMB AND BASMATI RICE

1 pound lean ground lamb
1 small onion, finely chopped
2 garlic cloves, pressed
1 tablespoon chopped cilantro
1 egg, beaten
Salt and freshly ground pepper to taste
2 tablespoons curry powder
1 cup chicken broth
1 cup tomato sauce
1 cup basmati rice, cooked

1. Combine lamb, onion, garlic, cilantro, egg, salt, and pepper in a large bowl. Mix thoroughly and form into meatballs.
2. Combine curry powder, broth, and tomato sauce in a saucepan or Dutch oven. Mix and heat to a simmer.
3. Add meatballs to sauce.
4. Cover and cook for forty-five minutes.
5. Serve with basmati rice.

SERVES: 4

LAMB, ZUCCHINI, AND MUSHROOM KEBABS

1 pound lean, cubed lamb, preferably from the leg
¼ cup dry red wine
2 tablespoons lime juice
1 garlic clove, pressed
1 tablespoon grated fresh ginger
¼ teaspoon cumin
¼ teaspoon hot pepper sauce
2 small zucchini, cut into 2-inch pieces
8 large mushroom caps

1. Place lamb cubes in a bowl.
2. Combine wine, lime juice, garlic, ginger, cumin, and hot pepper sauce. Mix thoroughly and pour over lamb.
3. Allow lamb to marinate for thirty minutes, turning meat in marinade every ten minutes.
4. Preheat oven to broil.
5. Thread lamb and vegetables on four skewers and place on a broiling pan. Pour remaining marinade over all.
6. Broil until lamb is browned and cooked to taste.

SERVES: 4

MONKFISH STEAKS IN ORANGE-GINGER SAUCE

2 teaspoons olive oil
1 red onion, sliced
3 garlic cloves, pressed
1 pound plum tomatoes, chopped
1 large seedless orange, peeled and coarsely chopped
2 tablespoons grated fresh ginger
Salt and freshly ground pepper to taste
4 monkfish steaks

1. Preheat oven to 350 degrees.
2. Heat oil in a large, nonstick skillet.
3. Add onion, garlic, tomatoes, orange, and ginger to skillet. Stir to combine.
4. Cover skillet and cook over low heat, stirring occasionally, for ten minutes. Season to taste.
5. Place fish steaks in a shallow baking pan. Pour sauce over fish.
6. Bake until fish is cooked through, about ten to twelve minutes.

SERVES: 4

QUICK MUSHROOM SOUP

¾ pounds mushrooms
4 cups low-sodium beef broth
Salt and freshly ground pepper to taste
1 tablespoon finely chopped flat or Italian parsley

1. Thinly slice mushrooms.
2. Combine mushrooms and broth in a saucepan. Cover and bring to a simmer. Cook over low heat for twenty minutes. Season.
3. Garnish soup with parsley.

SERVES: 4

NECTARINE RELISH

3 nectarines, coarsely chopped
2 firm tomatoes, coarsely chopped
3 green onions, finely chopped
½ teaspoon hot pepper sauce (or to taste)
1 tablespoon seasoned rice wine vinegar

1. Combine all ingredients in a bowl and mix thoroughly.
2. Chill for thirty minutes before serving.

YIELD: 2 CUPS

PEAR-GINGER SALAD

1 cup plain, low-fat yogurt
1 tablespoon grated fresh ginger
1 garlic clove, pressed
½ teaspoon Dijon mustard
4 large pears, peeled and diced
3 stalks celery, diced
2 cups chopped Romaine lettuce

1. Combine yogurt, ginger, garlic, and mustard. Mix
   well.
2. Place pears and celery in a large bowl. Add yogurt
   dressing and toss to combine.
3. Place chopped lettuce on a serving platter. Top with
   pear-ginger mixture.

SERVES: 4

PINEAPPLE FRUIT SALAD WITH GINGER-LIME DRESSING

1 fresh pineapple
1 cup raspberries
1 cup blueberries
1 cup melon balls
Ginger-Lime Dressing (see recipe on page 115)

1. Cut pineapple in half through the crown. Cut fruit out of each pineapple half.
2. Remove core and cut pineapple into chunks.
3. Combine pineapple with berries and melon balls. Mix and spoon back into pineapple shells.
4. Drizzle with Ginger-Lime Dressing.

SERVES: 4–6

PORK WITH GINGER AND VEGETABLES

2 teaspoons olive oil
1 pound pork tenderloin, cubed
2 tablespoons grated fresh ginger
2 garlic cloves, pressed
1 red bell pepper, thinly sliced
2 green onions, sliced
½ pound snow peas
1 cup cooked broccoli florets
1 teaspoon sesame oil

1. Heat oil in a large, nonstick skillet.
2. Add pork and brown lightly.
3. Add ginger, garlic, bell pepper, green onion, and snow peas. Saute over low heat, stirring frequently, for five minutes.
4. Add broccoli and sesame oil and stir to combine.
5. Cover and simmer until pork is cooked and all ingredients are heated through.

SERVES: 4

RAITA DIP FROM INDIA
FOR VEGETABLES

1 cup plain, low-fat yogurt
1 small cucumber, peeled, finely chopped
1 garlic clove, pressed
¼ teaspoon cumin (or to taste)
Pinch cayenne pepper

1. Combine all ingredients in a bowl. Mix thoroughly.
2. Refrigerate for thirty minute before serving with an assortment of raw vegetables.

YIELD: ABOUT 1½ CUPS

ROASTED RED PEPPERS AND SHRIMP

4 red bell peppers
1½ pounds large shrimp, cooked, shelled, and cleaned
2 tablespoons olive oil
1 tablespoon seasoned rice wine vinegar
1 garlic clove, pressed
2 green onions, thinly sliced
1 tablespoon flat or Italian parsley, finely chopped

1. Preheat oven to broil.
2. Place peppers in broiler pan in a single layer. Broil, turning peppers from side to side until they are charred.
3. Place peppers in a paper bag. Close bag and allow peppers to cool.
4. When peppers are cool enough to handle, scrape off charred skin. This is easily done under cold, running water.
5. Core and seed peppers, and cut each pepper into four slices.
6. Arrange peppers around perimeter of serving platter, and place shrimp in the center.
7. Combine oil, vinegar, and garlic, and mix thoroughly. Drizzle over peppers and shrimp.
8. Garnish with green onions and parsley.

SERVES: 4

SHRIMP AND SCALLOP CASSOULET

2 teaspoons olive oil
1 large onion, sliced
2 garlic cloves, chopped
2 red bell peppers, sliced
4 very ripe tomatoes, coarsely chopped
½ cup tomato juice
½ teaspoon red pepper flakes
   (optional)
Salt and freshly ground pepper to taste
½ cup cooked white beans
¾ pound medium shrimp, shelled
   and cleaned
½ pound sea scallops, cut in half

1. Heat oil in a large Dutch oven.
2. Add onion, garlic, bell peppers, tomatoes, and juice. Cover and cook over low heat until vegetables are thoroughly cooked and have combined into a sauce.
3. Add seasonings and beans.
4. Bring sauce to a simmer and add shrimp and scal-

lops. Cover and cook for about two minutes, or until seafood is just cooked. Be careful not to over-cook. Correct seasoning.

SERVES: 4

BAKED SALMON AND
CELERY CASSEROLE

*1 bunch celery, separated into stalks, trimmed, and cut
    in half*
2 cups chicken broth
1 tablespoon chopped flat or Italian parsley
1½ pounds fillet of salmon, cut into 4 slices
½ cup dry white wine
Salt and freshly ground pepper to taste

1. Place celery in a saucepan. Add broth and parsley. Cover and cook until celery is tender.
2. Preheat oven to 375 degrees.
3. Transfer celery and all liquid to a shallow, oven-proof casserole. Spread celery evenly in casserole.
4. Place salmon on top of celery bed, add wine, and season. Bake until salmon is cooked through.

SERVES: 4

FRENCH-STYLE TUNA SALAD

2 cups finely shredded red cabbage
1 cup finely shredded lettuce
2 red bell peppers, sliced into rings
2 tomatoes, quartered
4 green onions, thinly sliced
1 pound cooked tuna, cubed, or two 7-ounce cans solid
  white tuna, packed in water, drained
6 pitted black olives, sliced
Salt and freshly ground pepper to taste
Seasoned rice wine vinegar to taste

1. Combine cabbage and lettuce, and place around the perimeter of a serving platter.
2. Arrange pepper slices and tomatoes over cabbage-lettuce mixture. Sprinkle with green onion.
3. Place tuna in the center of the platter and top with black olives. Season.
4. Drizzle rice wine vinegar over all.

SERVES: 4

TURKEY LETTUCE WRAPS

2 teaspoons sesame oil
1 tablespoon light soy sauce
2 tablespoons grated fresh ginger
1 stalk celery, finely diced
4 red radishes, finely diced
4 green onions, thinly sliced
1 cup shredded cabbage
1 garlic clove, pressed
1 pound breast of turkey, finely diced
½ cup seasoned rice wine vinegar
1 teaspoon hot pepper sauce
1 teaspoon minced cilantro
1 head iceberg lettuce, separated into leaves

1. Combine oil, soy sauce, and ginger in a large, non-stick skillet, and cook over low heat for one minute.
2. Add celery, radish, green onion, cabbage, and garlic. Cover and cook until vegetables are just wilted. Transfer vegetable mixture to a large bowl.
3. Add turkey, vinegar, hot pepper sauce, and cilantro to skillet. Sauté, stirring, until turkey is cooked through, about five minutes.
4. Combine contents of skillet with vegetables and mix.

5. To serve: Present platter of lettuce leaves and turkey-vegetable mixture, and let everyone prepare their own wraps.

SERVES: 4

NINE

A Great Beginning

You've followed the Stop Smoking, Stay Skinny Program for thirty days, and you can see results. Maybe you've stopped smoking completely, and if you haven't, you know that you're on the way. Remember to look forward and not back. The past can't be changed, but the future can.

You have arrived at a life-affirming philosophy. This means that you like yourself enough to do the best for yourself. Sure, you liked smoking, but knowing that it's not in your best interest, you have been able to cut down or—hopefully—cut it out completely.

Perhaps you have not been as successful in stopping smoking as you had hoped. If so, you may be punishing yourself still further by continuing to do the wrong thing. Try to understand the emotions that are driving you into a potentially destructive situation. You need relief from the inner pressures that push you in that direction so that you can fulfill yourself instead of destroying yourself.

Think of the Program as something to follow one day at a time—it's easier to say, "I won't smoke for the next twenty-four hours," than to think you'll never smoke again.

Stop thinking of a cigarette as a reward. Smoking is just a substitute for a *real reward*—the reward of feeling great and knowing that you have a long life to look forward to.

THE ABILITY TO CHANGE

One of the things the Stop Smoking, Stay Skinny Program does is to assess your capacity for change. You may have discovered a wonderful ability: You are open to new ideas—you're not in a rut. Change can be constructive, you realize, something to enjoy rather than to fear. Today you can say proudly, "I've stopped smoking," and tomorrow that newly discovered ability may impact beneficially on your relationships and career.

Congratulations and welcome to the rest of your life.

INDEX

F

Fat in foods, low fat/no fat foods, 60–61
Fats
  and L-carnitine, 17–18
  and lecithin, 19
Fish, recommended types, 51
Fish/seafood recipes
  fisherman's chowder, 112
  fish fillets, stuffed, with gingersauce, 110–111
  gazpacho with scallops, 114
  monkfish steaks, in orange-ginger sauce, 120
  salmon and celery casserole, 130
  shrimp and roasted red peppers, 127
  shrimp and scallop cassoulet, 128
  tuna salad, French-style, 131
Five-Step Plan, 23–34
  listening in, 24–25
  reorienting, 24, 29–31
  stopping, 24, 26–27
  switching, 24, 28–29

G

DR. JOSEPH T. MARTORANO has been in private practice in psychiatry for over twenty-five years. He has been on the faculty of major teaching hospitals in New York and is an expert in psychopharmacology. Coauthor of two highly successful books, *Beyond Negative Thinking* and *Unmasking PMS,* Dr. Martorano is a nationally recognized authority on the clinical treatment of PMS, and is cofounder and medical director of PMS Medical.

CARMEL BERMAN REINGOLD has published more than twenty-five books, many dealing with health and diet. Her popular *The Lifelong Anti-Cancer Diet* appeared in Japanese and Portuguese editions, and she was featured on Japanese as well as American television. A well-known food writer, Ms. Reingold authored *California Cuisine* and coauthored *Cooking with David Burke.* A former contributing editor at *Woman* magazine, she has written for *Bride's* and *Cosmopolitan,* as well as other publications.

Complete and Authoritative
Health Care Sourcebooks
from Avon Books

EMERGENCY CHILDCARE:
A Pediatrician's Guide   by Peter T. Greenspan M.D.
77635-9/$5.99 US/$7.99 Can   and Suzanne Le Vert

A HANDBOOK OF NATURAL
FOLK REMEDIES   by Elena Oumano Ph. D.
78448-3/$5.99 US/$7.99 Can

ESTROGEN: **Answers to**
All Your Questions   by Mark Stolar, M.D.
79076-9/$5.99 US/$7.99 Can

MIGRAINES: **Everything You**
Need to Know About Their
Cause and Cure   by Arthur Elkind, M.D.
79077-7/$5.99 US/$7.99 Can

HGH: **The Promise of**
Eternal Youth   by Suzanne Le Vert
78885-3/$5.99 US/$7.99 Can

HELP AND HOPE FOR
HAIR LOSS   by Gary S. Hitzig, M.D.
78710-5/$6.50 US/$8.50 Can

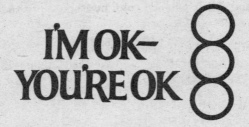

Expertly detailed, pharmaceutical guides
can now be at your fingertips
from U.S. Pharmacopeia

THE USP GUIDE TO MEDICINES
78092-5/$6.99 US/$8.99 Can

- More than 2,000 entries for both prescription
  and non-prescription drugs
- Handsomely detailed color insert

THE USP GUIDE
TO HEART MEDICINES
78094-1/$6.99 US/$8.99 Can

- Side effects and proper dosages for over 400
  brand-name and generic drugs
- Breakdown of heart ailments such as angina,
  high cholesterol and high blood pressure

THE USP GUIDE TO
VITAMINS AND MINERALS
78093-3/$6.99 US/$8.99 Can

- Precautions for children, senior citizens and
  pregnant women
- Latest findings and benefits of dietary supplements